D1233564

WHY
MOVEMENT
IS
MEDICINE

Dr. Cuan Coetzee DC

ISBN: 979-8-69-326987-3
Imprint: Independently published

First editor: Neil Le Roux
Second editor: Kerry Vice

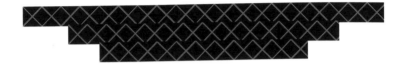

First printing edition 2020.

@cuan33 | g.page/cuan33

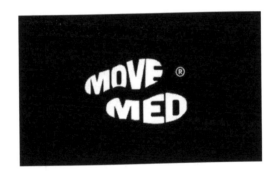

Dedication

To my family.

Dad, Mom, Kay, Nix, Cam and Scott.

To everyone else.

Yes, you. For making the first small move.

Eyewitnesses

Cuan is an enigma; an unexpected breath of fresh air in any environment - he is always the most positive, passionate and persuasive man in the room. I would be surprised if anyone cares as much about your physical and emotional health as the author of "Why Movement Is Medicine". What makes this book so special and significant is not the wealth of knowledge and information it contains, but the nature of its creator - someone who lives it, and lives to empower others to live it too! - Mark Paul

Cuan is the most generous person I know. This book is a gift of his knowledge to help you live your healthiest life. What better gift could one receive? - Nicole Coetzee

Cuan is a master in his field. He always made sure he keeps on top of things. He gives his all to all of our patients and has great results. He is caring and passionate in not only his work but in life as well. His knowledge is impeccable. I am grateful to have worked closely with him and proud to call him my friend. - Dr Jason Thoresen (MD)

Dr Cuan Coetzee is one of those professionals that I could always confidently refer my patients to, as I knew he was not only an excellent chiropractor who would manage their medical conditions well, but he is also an exceptional human being who used his God given talents to inspire and encourage people to live healthier more balanced lives. - Dr Eljoh Lombard (MD)

Dr Cuan Coetzee is unquestionably the embodiment of someone who practices what they preach. A true master in movement, with a depth of knowledge and intellect one very rarely encounters in life - a salubrious genius. - Dr Quinton Hohls (DC)

Being fortunate enough to call Cuan one of my closest

friends, I am aware of the time and effort that went into this book. There is no half measure when it comes to Cuan: he adds and contributes with everything he does. I know many people will benefit from this book. I have. - Dr Lochner Slabbert (DC)

From the streets of East London to the boroughs of London, Cuan is making his mark and crowds are chanting his mantra and getting moving - 'Otherwise, you well?' – Dr Robyn Spring (MD)

Preface

My name is Dr Cuan Coetzee. I believe that life is a gift. It should never be taken for granted. I mean, it is dreamlike that for a living I have the privilege of potentially altering the trajectory of someone's life.

That all changed the day before yesterday. I nearly killed someone.

Forewords

Chad le Clos

(London Olympic Games 2012 Gold Medallist)

I met Cuan briefly for the first time in 2012. However, it was only a year later at the 2013 FINA World Championships trials in Port Elizabeth that I got to know him a little more. I remember that he went out of his way, while on holiday, to give me a massage and a rubdown before that evening's finals competition.

It was there that I learnt that we have a few things in common - our family means everything to us, hard work always pays off and within your field of expertise you can do anything you put your mind to.

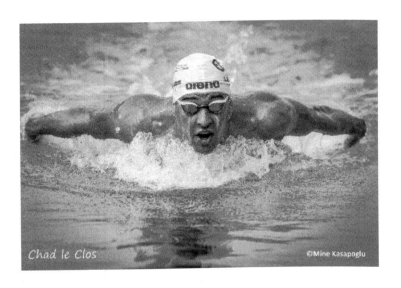

Chad le Clos

©Mine Kasapoglu

Anaso Jobodwana

(IAAF World Championships 2015 Bronze Medallist)

As a wide-eyed grade eight pupil, I grew up looking up to Cuan. He was a leader of the school and he had a positive energy which he put into all his work; both in the classroom and on the track. So years later, when I would visit home, it was only natural that I went to him for my therapy sessions. Of course, I was not disappointed. He is attentive, thorough, and very dedicated to his work, making sure that I came out of his office with a healthy body.

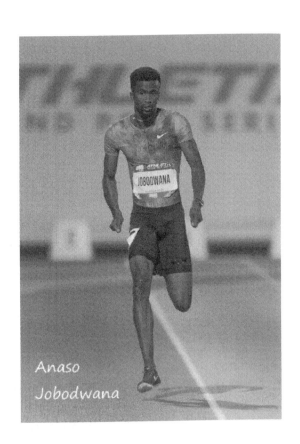

Anaso
Jobodwana

Prologue

I grew up learning that you must be hospitable. If people come and see you, you offer them something. In my job, people come and see me, and I need to offer them something more than a beverage, more than treatment for the cause of their pain. I choose education. A little bit of pain relief and preventing years of dysfunction in their bodies, (and ultimately morbidity), is a bonus.

I also grew up learning that you must always be prepared for any circumstance. Both miracles and disasters take no reservations. For some people, a loaf of bread gifted is a miracle, and others a cancer in remission. For some, a headache is a disaster, and others a death in the family. I have learnt that these examples are all valid, as your experience is relative to you as an individual.

In my experience of the conservative primary health care industry, I have become fed up with the enormity of substandard health care across the board. Substandard in terms of the number of patients becoming dependent on drugs and medications and leaving paid consultations with no new knowledge about their condition or how to prevent their problems from recurring. The purpose of this book is to enlighten you about some of the ways to lower your risk of chronic diseases, to improve your quality of life and to educate you about many day-to-day ailments that I have witnessed which can easily be prevented.

I have the privilege of being a Health Coach and Chiropractor[1]. For a living I identify movement irregularities in people that lead to the degeneration of the spine and body and we formulate a plan to prevent the progression of this degeneration. In turn, people have less pain, are often happier because of it and can perform the activities of daily living that they were not able to do before. My job is addictive, even euphoric. People are excited when they see me. The fact that patients can move, bend, sit, sleep or perform normal body functions easier or better than before. That is worth getting excited about.

I would love it if after reading this book you are inspired in *some* way to start *some* form of exercise and incorporate *some* form of dietary changes. If you are already involved in exercise and healthy eating, I hope this book shows you how to truly amplify the benefits of those. My hope is to reintroduce these to you over the next few chapters.

What I am going to tell you in the upcoming chapters may change your life, or it may not, but something as simple as getting moving or changing a bad habit may be what you need to make a small positive change in your life. This in turn has the potential to alter your future or the futures of those around you. And let me tell you: I would rather watch paint dry than watch someone not reach their full health potential.

I have been a student, an intern, an associate, a locum and the owner of a practice. A good portion of this book is about my life, and some of the experiences that have literally shaped and moulded my mind, my body and my spirit. It is also an account of how I came to grips with how our lifestyles impact on our ability to be alive, whether we like it or not.

---

[1] Or *fake doctor* as I have heard before. My brother is an orthopaedic surgeon, so I will happily claim the name *fake doctor* in comparison to him. But the reality is that anyone referred to as a doctor is merely a teacher, that is what the word doctor means. I reckon that anyone who is not educating their patients should not be called a doctor in the first place. Enough spoilers for now, let's read on.

Ideas started brewing for this book way back when I was teenager. Now complete, I am aged 31 and living under 'lockdown' due to the Covid 19 Pandemic. The point is that everything is always changing, even if we do not always notice it. Nothing is set in stone[2]. Your life can be made or lost in a matter of seconds. All we can do is control what we can control. And this book is full of things that you *can* control.

So here are the rules:

I do not have a clue what any of you are going through. I never grew up in your home. I never knew your parents. I do not even know if you are physically able to move. I am only an expert on how to be me – on what has helped and changed my life.

Please note, the contents of this book, regardless of implication, and the statements expressed herein are not intended to be a substitute for direct professional medical advice.

Some statements or statistics may have come from things I have experienced, picked up, read in articles or heard from colleagues or other professionals. Some statements may be impossible to reference individually, but their input has shaped the way my thought processes have developed and therefore I am incredibly grateful.

All patients' names have been changed and substituted with names from well-known TV series or movies, for obvious confidentiality reasons. I like my job, and I do not particularly want to be barred from doing it by the fun police[3].

---

[2] Except for an epitaph (the writing that goes on your tombstone one day if you do not donate your body to science). That is pretty much set in stone. By the way, I think you should consider donating your body to science, or, at the very least donate your organs. You could save a life or let a medical / chiropractic student cut you open - either/or.

[3] This idea came from the master, Adam Kay. Also, the idea for this type of footnote throughout the book came from his *best-seller THIS IS GOING TO HURT*. It is only fitting that he gets one the first few footnotes.

The first example of one of my patient's cases is that of Jon Snow. Jon's case will appear at the beginning of each chapter. Each part of his case may not relate to the contents of that chapter, but it is an interesting case that you can follow throughout the book. Spoiler, it ends strangely in chapter 21.

Any of my opinions (the first footnote as one example) which go against the grain are not meant to give offence, nor are they meant to criticise any individuals or industries. They are merely the observations that I have made, using my training and my experience.

These are my personal experiences. Everything that my patients and I have tried and tested. My aim is to discuss health principles in a way that *anyone* would also be able to follow. So, stand back, relax and enjoy the read.

I would say *sit* back but sitting is literally the worst thing you can do to yourself. *Sitting is the new smoking.*

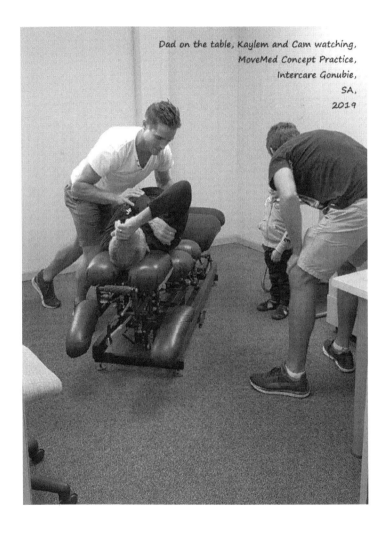

Dad on the table, Kaylem and Cam watching,
MoveMed Concept Practice,
Intercare Gonubie,
SA,
2019

1 : Moving Medicine

Jon Snow, a 33-year-old bastard, presents to the clinic. Jon was referred by an existing patient. *This is always a great start. Patient is now expectant of an accurate diagnosis and hopefully some quick results.*

I f you were wondering about my role in nearly killing someone, I mean I never educated him enough about the first step to changing his life. Towards the end of the book you will learn what that first step is. After all if you are not busy living, and constantly improving your health, you are dying.

A genetic metabolic neurologist was famously quoted in THE TIMES magazine as saying, "If there was a drug that could do for human health everything that exercise can, it would likely be the most valuable pharmaceutical ever developed".

Preach.

One way to view good health is to see it as merely the slowest possible rate at which you can die. The reality is that being healthy means having an internal healing environment. It is a seesaw tilting in that favour. This is what I have observed in my clinical and personal life. Before you can heal, you need to ask yourself if you are willing to give up the things that made you ill in the first place. That is the first step in the healing process - a conscious choice. Do not look your health gift horse in the mouth. If you have good health, maintain it. If you do not, now is the time to start helping your body to heal itself.

One of my hopes and desires for this book is that you will see what movement, exercise, clean eating and quality recovery has done for my life - how they have transformed me physically, emotionally, chemically, psychologically and spiritually, and how or why they could do the same for you. These are truths for me. Hopefully, they can become truths for you too. So, take them, use them, share them, copy them. They are yours for free if you choose them[4].

When we hear the word movement, exercise is often the first thing that pops into our minds. But in this context movement could mean one of many things. This move in the right direction could be as simple as a conscious choice to want to make a change. This is the most important first move.

---

[4] Spiritually. In my experiences, this is the most significant aspect of a patient's health journey. You need to want to help yourself. You need to be expectant about getting better. And that speaks into belief. It does not matter what you believe in, but I think it is fair to assume that part of the process of health and healing is a belief in getting better. A belief in someone, something, the process, the practitioner, or the practice. Let us focus on these in the upcoming chapters. We know that belief is relative to the individual. For me, rather than meditating on the opinions of people on social media, on the daily commentaries of the rich and famous, or the so called news that the media bombard us with (all of which follow a moral philosophy of some sort because they are all full of judgment), I have chosen to believe in Jesus. I have chosen to meditate on a moral philosophy as old as time. And FYI, no part of this book is suggestive of any belief as the perceived right choice.

The rest: optimism, exercise, clean eating, psychosocial and spiritual wholeness, and possibly even happiness, will all fall into place.

Time really does fly, but I never expected the truth to be so literal. Time seems to pass by ever so quickly. And such is life. Before we know it, we are in our golden years and then it is all over. Everybody dies. It is the one thing all humans can be relied on to do well. Yet it still comes as a surprise to some people. One of the ways I know to make life count is through the pursuit of health.

It is impossible for me to give one program that fits all. Or one diet. Or one eating pattern. There are no quick fixes to be in good health. What we need is to start moving better and moving more. We need to prioritize healthy habits and this book is full of guidance as to what these are. I tell my patients that it is better for you to decide for yourself when you want to retire, as opposed to your body forcing you into retirement. Take back the control.

It is human nature that most of us will resist change. Most people fight change as if change is worse than that which they are experiencing. When you look to the future, you must believe and know without doubt that you can reform fundamental habits, that you can change, that you have genius in you, goodness in you and perseverance in you.

I have witnessed many secrets of the human body: how it responds to treatments, what it looks like when you cut it open, and just how intricate it is. But one truth about our bodies is that among all else, the body is a material object - it is easily torn, and not easily mended.

We all have our teeth, blood pressure, cholesterol, blood sugar and eyes checked regularly, yet somehow, we forget to have our brains checked as often. By brain in this context, I mean the part of the brain we can manually assist, i.e. the spinal nerves which the brain uses to communicate with every tissue in the body. The crux of the matter is that if the signals about an area of the body are not getting to the brain in the first place, (and therefore adequate quality responses are not elicited), then healing cannot happen. That is where I come in[5]. My goal is to remove any physical irritation to the nervous system, and, to give advice and education about how to limit chemical and emotional irritations. An entire chapter is devoted to this issue later.

Remove, re-move, move.

We need to get our bodies moving the way they were designed to move. *'Remove'* means eradicating stressors that prevent the body from healing itself. *'Re-move'* means emphasizing the need to re-educate the body about how it is designed to move after an abnormal movement pattern has developed from an unrehabilitated injury. *'Move'* speaks to the need to maintain movement and to develop a positive and efficient movement pattern that will prevent physical body wear and tear in the future.

Here is an example[6].

March 2016

Ray Romano, a 36-year-old male patient, presents to the clinic. He is a bumbling well-intentioned father that everybody loves.

He presents with an acute (less than 3 days) onset of low

---

[5] Or any chiropractor, really. The way I practice is called *mixed* chiropractic. More specifically, it is health coaching. Whatever we need to do to satisfy the patients' health needs, we do. That includes physical treatment and helping the patient manage any risk factors that they present with. More on this in the chapters *Healing, Pain* and *the F-Word*.

[6] Welcome to the first of the cases. To prevent utter boredom, I am only going to present the main symptoms, conditions we have seen before that we needed to rule out, and the single most beneficial treatment that we performed. Treatments would normally include most of the following: MoveMed NRE protocol, chiropractic adjustments, myofascial release, trigger point needling, stretching, heat application and specific rehabilitation exercises.

back pain. *No history of low back pain before this, only stiffness, for roughly 10 years, along with sciatica (the odd electric shock shooting down his leg). No history of motor vehicle accidents or trauma reported.*

We ruled out Baastrup's disease (also known as Kissing spine syndrome). Kissing Spine is a disease where the spaces between the back of the vertebrae reduce and the vertebrae touch, or 'kiss', causing bone-to-bone contact.

X-rays were justified and taken, and Ray displayed severe spinal degeneration in both his neck and lumbar spine. His diagnosis was severe disc degeneration and intervertebral foramen encroachment as a result of the degenerative changes (the spine is beginning to crumble and change shape - most likely from years of poor posture).

Ray responded to a Neural Re-Education protocol and managed his back with monthly checks. Everybody still loves him.

The good-to-knows:

ONE. These spinal changes happen over a minimum of fifteen years and they are not normal for his age[7]. If he had not responded to conservative treatment, a neurosurgeon would have needed to have been consulted.

TWO. Patient had NO significant pain prior to this episode.

THREE. Without management, Romano's spinal prognosis was poor.

---

[7] You always feel better when your doctor says your condition is normal for your age, but you do realise that dying will also be normal for your age eventually. Not so?

This is one of many cases in point. Had he known what risk factors or warning signs to look out for, it could have been prevented. Had he known about simple spine biomechanics and how the body is meant to move, the situation could possibly have been prevented. Had someone taken the time to ask him the correct questions or give him some advice, it could possibly have prevented this case. Had he been informed what exercise is beneficial for his body and spine, I would bet money that most of his problems could have been prevented[8].

Neural Re-Education (NRE) is something that we have tried and tested for many years now and we have seen remarkable results in practice. Fingers crossed there is a clinical trial pending. There is a lot on NRE in the upcoming chapters. To understand what makes exercise so great, we need to understand how it affects the brain and how it helps the body develop new neural connections, NRE. If your brain has only become used to pain, we need to teach it what normal feels like again. This is one of the ways that help alleviate pain.

In the media, exercise and diet are both often superficially marketed. Typically, the main benefits are touted as being heart health and weight loss. While these are still good for you, less is said about the real benefits of movement and clean eating; things like increased muscle mass, longer healthy years of life, less insulin sensitivity, fewer links with depression and anxiety, and anti-inflammatory effects.

There are questions that are often posed to me during consultations. *How can I stay healthy for longer? Why is my pain not going away? What is the single most beneficial thing I can do for my spine?* We all have different priorities. The

---

[8] This is one of the themes I want you to take away from this book. Education is everything. You need to leave a consultation knowing more than when you arrived. Prevention is better than cure, every time. This is one of the many truths in medicine, but one often not emphasized. I always say: if your doctor has not touched you, or educated you, you are not seeing a doctor - you are seeing a businessman.

question I pose to myself is, *how can I run for the rest of my life?*

The answers to all these questions are: *KEEP ON MOVING.* And: *EAT CLEAN.* You do not have to be an exercise enthusiast or a professional athlete, you just need to start somewhere. Move one muscle, one ligament or one joint at a time. If you are not moving, just start moving. If you are exercising already, keep it up.

From my clinical experience, if exercise could be purchased in the form of a pill, it would be the single most widely prescribed and beneficial medicine in the world. At the end of this chapter lookout for the x-ray of a patient who has had a spinal fusion. You can clearly see all the metalwork. Spinal operations, spinal disc injuries, headaches and low back pain are the most common conditions I treat and manage in private practice, and most of them are treatable and are often preventable. Even better, most of the treatment is free. If we could try and move the way we were designed to move, the spine and the body would look after themselves.

So how can this help you? For one thing, let us try and avoid ever needing a spinal fusion.

In around 450 BC, the Father of Medicine, Hippocrates, said that all parts of the body if unused and left idle will become liable to disease, defective in growth and will age quickly. You see, it seems that medicine at its core, is movement.

So, when did that all change?

Most patients come to me because they are in pain. Please understand that that is the *worst* time to consult someone. Pain is often the last symptom to present itself and it is almost always the easiest to treat, but it is a poor indicator of the underlying degeneration that is happening in the body and spine. The time is now, get moving.

I remember reading somewhere that if you want to make everyone happy, do not become an educator. Instead, sell ice-cream. Well I disagree. We will not live forever but while we are alive, we can live well. For me, as a doctor, that is what I want to see. Is there an area of your life where you would like to improve? If you look to the future, would you change that one thing? Is exercise that area? Is your diet that area? Then the time is now.

Let's go.

Point to ponder: In what area within your life can you make the first small change?

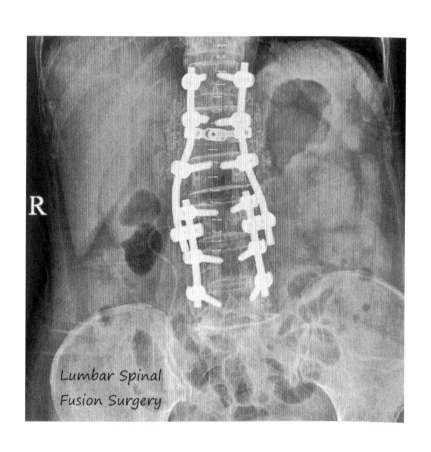

R

Lumbar Spinal
Fusion Surgery

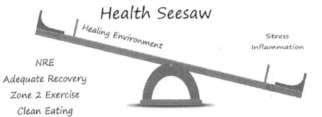

Health Seesaw

Healing Environment

Stress
Inflammation

NRE
Adequate Recovery
Zone 2 Exercise
Clean Eating
Positive Mindset

2 : Moving New York

Jon has severe, debilitating, acute low back pain following an incident lifting a fridge. Two-day onset. Pain 9/10. Patient describes "sharp, burning and shooting" pain into his right leg, calf and under the foot. *Excellent, something is clearly hitting that L5 nerve.*

I never really had the desire to run a road marathon. I always thought it was silly and, to be honest, a bit excessive. You do not need to finish a marathon to prove that you can run. That was until I was offered the opportunity to run a marathon. The ultimate marathon. Through the streets of the greatest city in the world. Little did I know that it would turn out to be one of the most exhilarating things I could do in my lifetime.

This stage of learning is called: Accept the challenge.

Eliud Kipchoge. If you have not heard his name until now,

he is the greatest male marathoner to date. The Kenyan runner has topped the podium in 11 of his 13 marathon races over 42.2 km. He is the current Olympic champion and holds the world record for the distance: 2:01:39 set in Berlin.

On October 12, 2019, he went one step further by becoming the first person ever to run under two hours for a marathon. At a special time-trial event in Vienna, Eliud completed the 42.2 km distance in 1:59:40. He broke one of distance running's final big hurdles. The run could be compared to visiting the moon and returning to Earth, or the first summit of Everest[9].

It is therefore worth pausing and considering how ridiculously fast this run is. Let me break it down. It is around 4:34.5 per mile for each of the 26 miles, or under a 2:50 min/km pace for 42 kilometres. At no point did he fall behind the targeted 1:59:59 pace.

To put this into context, Eliud would have to repeatedly run 28:26 for every 10km. Or think of it this way, he had to run 100m sprints in just over 17 seconds, 422 times in a row. This is unbelievable. Those figures might not mean much when they are viewed on their own, but when compared to the pace at which we mere mortals run, they are ludicrous.

Challenges are relative, and so for me 2:59 was the goal. I would attempt to run under three hours in my first road marathon.

---

[9] I recommend going onto YouTube and watching the last kilometre of this run. Anyone, of any age, would appreciate it. I cry almost every time. He had teams of pacemakers helping him, who on any other day would be his rivals, and to see how ecstatic they all are for him that he finally broke this barrier is stirring. Like Michael Phelps's 4x100m relay team that helped him secure one of his eight gold medals at the Beijing Games. Phelps's teammate Jason Lezak's final leg comeback chasing the then world record holder is often considered to be the greatest swim the sport has ever seen. This speaks to the power of living for something greater than yourself.

New York

In June 2019 I was offered a charity spot to run the New York City marathon, arguably the best rated marathon in the world. It was a chance to run through some of the most iconic scenes in the movie business as well as all five boroughs of New York City. The start is on Staten Island, also known as the 'Forgotten Borough'. Not much happens there. The second borough is Brooklyn, which is my second favourite place after Cintsa[10]. The third borough is Queens, home of the New York Mets and the fourth is The Bronx, home of the New York Yankees. The finish is in the fifth borough, Manhattan, the heart of The Big Apple.

I instantly grabbed it with both hands. The charity was the Zara Centre for AIDS Impacted Youth in Bulawayo, Zimbabwe. It is a cause that is geographically and emotionally close to home. One of our domestic helpers, with whom we grew up, had passed away from HIV, and we knew so many others in our local community who had also succumbed. The effects of this dreaded disease on families, especially in Southern Africa, is a very real one.

Being the competitive person that I am, I instantly wanted to break three hours for the race. This was for a few other reasons over and above wanting to be in the top 2% of the running world. In 2017, the winner of the New York Marathon ran 2:10. Of the 50641 runners that year, 35654 ran under five hours, 14024 ran under four and only 1092 runners ran under three hours.

In the marathon running world, the sub-three-hour running time sets you up as an above-average runner. It is a holy grail of sorts for amateur athletes or age groupers (people with full time jobs).

Another motivator was my brother. 'Sub 3' was something

---

[10] I will elaborate on Cintsa later but for now just know that it is a small stretch of paradise on the South African East Coast.

that my brother had tried to accomplish twice in marathons and both times he had just missed it. His times were 3.03 and 3.08. My brother is still the most talented runner I personally know[11].

In 2018, the winner of the New York Marathon ran a time of 2.05. Of the 52706 runners that year, 36328 ran under five, 14442 ran under four and 1206 runners ran under three hours. Again, only 2% of the runners ran 'Sub-3'.

Challenge accepted.

The race was two months away from when I heard I had an entry, and I luckily had a relatively good base-fitness having just completed the London Duathlon. By 'base' I mean I ran on average 160km per month from May to August. Even though this is typically low mileage for marathoners, it would have to suffice for a heavy runner[12]. Nick Bester, a competitive runner who you will meet later, runs 160km per week in his marathon training blocks, but he is superhuman in my books.

---

[11] Kaylem Coetzee. My one and only brother, my best friend, amazing father, loving husband and second favourite son in our family. Also, at present, the second fastest runner in our family and an orthopaedic surgeon. Kaylem taught me that any circumstance in life, no matter how desperate it may seem at the time, can be overcome. There is more about him, his own family, and our lives together throughout this book.

[12] I weigh 82kg. This has been my functional weight for the last ten years. Something you must always remember, is that you will have your own personal functional weight. If you go over this weight, (which is obesity), you will have health problems. If you are constantly trying to stay under your functional weight, you will have health problems. And this is the problem caused by years of fitness and fashion models being on covers of magazines. They have aesthetically good-looking bodies which may not necessarily be all that functional.

In 2018, *Strava*[13] had released statistics from over 10 000 runners who completed the London Marathon. This information revealed that as an average, the sub-three-hour marathon runners trained roughly twice as much (in terms of the distance run and the number of runs) as those who ran sub-four-hour marathons. Basically, most sub-three-hour marathon athletes were running 100km a week over eight runs, compared to my 50km a week over four runs, for a few months.

According to this I was solidly in the four-hour marathon group in terms of distance run per month, which was not a good start. Most coaches I had spoken to said that I needed to have run 100km per week, for a period of months to years, to have the endurance capability to run a 'Sub 3'.

The odds really were stacked up against me. As I was nowhere near those numbers, my thoughts at that stage were again, *challenge accepted*.

My strategy was to fine tune the training, working on becoming efficient, remaining healthy, and becoming comfortable "turning myself inside out". That was always the saying I used when competing in my school days. It was my mantra.

Another strategy was *Neural Re-Education*. This is one of the themes of this book. In theory, you need to teach the *brain* how to run. The brain controls the muscles and joints that you use when you run. Consequently, when you get tired during a race, the brain takes over, like the autopilot in an aeroplane, and your body will hold your running form. There is a way to

---

[13] Strava is an internet service for tracking exercise. It is mostly used for cycling and running using GPS data. As you finish your exercise, the details of your activity (such as your route, distance, elevation, time, average speed, heart rate etc.) gets posted onto your timeline. It is basically social media for exercise activities. And as with social media, we mostly use it in an attempt to attain more *likes*.

teach the brain to do this, and it is called 'Zone 2 Running'[14].

I realised that my longest road run before the race would be around 30km, so the last 12km of the marathon would be new territory for me, and new territory in sport always means you will need mental toughness. How comfortable can you remain while the body is screaming at you and various functions begin to shut down?

I included regular chiropractic adjustments, physically and physiologically keeping the joints of my body moving effectively. The body is a biological and living machine, and there are simple biomechanics that are identical in property to those of a machine. Efficiently moving parts in a machine means less friction. Less friction means less energy is needed to keep the cogs turning. This means less wear and tear (which can cause rust). If you try and move a rusty door hinge you will get the idea. In the body, less friction means less inflammation; less inflammation symptomatically means less pain, but more importantly less inflammation means less scar tissue development and reduces the risk of arthritis[15].

---

[14] There is a lot more on these phenomena later in the book. A quick spoiler, you do not need to run fast all the time, or exercise like Rocky every attempt you get, to get fitter, faster or healthier. Most times, the opposite is true.

[15] I am often told by people, like the stereotypical *know-it-all* on Facebook, that marathons kill your knee cartilage and *everyone* who does them is going to get arthritis. My first response is: *look at the research, the opposite is true*. My second response is: *it is not the race itself that will cause long term cartilage damage, it is the hundreds of hours of training*. Especially if you are not training smart. If you train smart, Zone 2 smart, and prioritize your full recovery after sessions, in my critical and clinical opinion, you can train for the rest of your life. More on this later.

Now if the research said I was meant to be running 100km per week for months to years to have the endurance capability of a 'Sub 3', why even try my 2:59 challenge?[16].

Firstly, the numbers did not account for genetics. Everyone is unique, so it is not always the case that if you run long distances you are going to succeed in running Sub-3. That was merely the majority. Secondly, the numbers also did not account for experience, or in my case, lack of marathon running experience. Before this, I had only completed one marathon and that was off-road, on trails. It included an elevation gain of approximately 2800m, and a few river crossings. Compared to a road race, it is run at a much slower pace of five hours. It is an entirely different bag of tricks compared to flat out tar pounding for three hours[17].

The one thing I did have experience in was years of treating marathon runners. Marathon runners love to hurt themselves. I was always able to pick their brains and observe how the injuries happened and what the risk factors were[18].

Now if I did not need to be a professional marathon runner, an experienced marathon runner, nor a 100km-a-week athlete, what did I need to do to attain this elusive marathon time of 2:59? What would I need to do to make it into the top 2% of marathon runners? I knew I needed to get used to at least 100km a week for a few weeks, but I also needed to do some speed work. It was going to be tricky.

---

[16] When interpreting research, it is always crucial to determine the quality and the context of the research. You need to become Walter White (the highly intelligent chemist from the TV series Breaking Bad) and break bad science. I did not think of myself as the average runner, so why rely on average research? I try to discredit many common misconceptions in this book.

[17] The Otter Trail, the most famous hiking trail in South Africa, opens its access once a year for the African Otter Trail Marathon. If you are ever visiting South Africa, and if the Otter trail is near your desired destination, I highly recommend it.

[18] I also had some physiological knowledge from a master's degree, an international sports course, and a few years of clinical experience.

So here it goes. This was my eight-week 2:59 challenge plan.

First, let us back up to the 8th of September, the London Duathlon. This race went exactly as planned and I managed to place third. It took just over two hours of racing which included 44km of cycling and 15km of running, so I knew I had some form in my legs. This race did come at a small price, unfortunately; in pushing hard at the beginning I had picked up a niggle during the race, a grade one calf strain. I knew it needed two weeks of TLC[19] before any marathon training could continue. New York was eight weeks away. It was game on! I like to be practical; it was time to do some maths. The equation and thought process ahead looked as follows.

(8 weeks to race) – (2 weeks TLC and MoveMed rehabilitation) = 6 weeks to race.

(6 weeks to race) – (3 weeks of zone 2 *big* distance) = 3 weeks to race.

(3 weeks to race) – (10 days of speed endurance) = 11 days of taper to race day.

It really would be touch and go. I could not afford to get sick, or pick up an injury, or allow my calf niggle to get worse. Therefore, the essential addition to this plan would be quality recovery. Quality recovery (you will see later) means sufficient sleep, making time to sleep, listening to my resting heart rate and clean eating. I did not want to place additional stress on my body. The only stress would be work and the stress of training. These were non-negotiable for me.

My Garmin fitness tracking device logged every session,

---

[19] Tender love and care. Also known as treatment. I have observed a trend at social gatherings. When people hear that I am a chiropractor, they always instantly and conveniently have a *stiff neck*, or they ask me to *quickly adjust* them. That is why I always hold a glass of wine. I can then explain that I do not treat after I have had something to drink. It is a great excuse. Works most times.

both running and cross training, as well as resting heart rate and sleep hours. Here is how the two-month block went, day by day, all the way up to race day. This was the first time I had kept such a rigid training diary, and the transformation was remarkable to witness. Here is my training journal for the eight weeks building up to the marathon. Notice: no running for the first two weeks[20].

---

[20] Learn to be patient, or you may become one. This is one of my favourite sayings in health. This applies to life in general too. On numerous occasions I have learnt that *haste makes waste*. I once ate an entire bowl of hamster muesli whilst visiting Kaylem and Nicole in Port Elizabeth. In my hastiness, I assumed that the hamster on the front packaging was the muesli's mascot.

Phase One (Recovery after London Duathlon)

Monday	60 min rehab [21]	Average resting HR: 51
Tuesday	60 min rehab	
Wednesday	60 min rehab	
Thursday	60 min rehab	
Friday	60 min rehab	
Saturday	75 min rehab and 20km cycle[22]	
Sunday	REST	Average resting HR: 52
Monday	45 min rehab and 20km cycle	
Tuesday	90 min rehab	
Wednesday	60 min rehab	
Thursday	60 min rehab	
Friday	60 min rehab	
Saturday	60 min rehab	

---

[21] A typical MoveMed rehabilitation exercise session incorporates Core, Proprioception and Flexibility exercises, usually in the form of interval training. There are chapters on all of these to look forward to. An example would be a 30 x one minute routine where every minute is a new exercise ranging from core activation to proprioception balance exercises to functional active stretching. You can start with 10 or 20 minutes. Remember, baby steps. You can refer to my YouTube channel for these.

[22] Cycling is mostly safe for a calf strain, as it incorporates concentric muscle activations, as opposed to eccentric calf contractions during the landing phase of a running stride. Fancy words, I know. The first phrase means 'shortening muscle' while the latter means 'lengthening muscle'.

Phase Two (Zone 2 100km Per Week Distance[23])

Sunday	20km run	Average resting HR: 53
Monday	REST	
Tuesday	18km run (with 8 x 1 minute at 3.45m/km)	
Wednesday	30km run	
Thursday	REST	
Friday	21km run	
Saturday	10km run	
Sunday	REST	Average resting HR: 52
Monday	25km run (morning 40min 10km at 4m/km, afternoon 15km zone2)	
Tuesday	25km run	
Wednesday	REST	
Thursday	21km run	
Friday	22km run	
Saturday	11km run	
Sunday	REST	Average resting HR: 52
Monday	25km run (with 12 x 1km at 4m/km)	
Tuesday	15km run	
Wednesday	REST	
Thursday	10km run	
Friday	30km run	
Saturday	20km run	

---

[23] Here is it again. Zone 2 is strictly the pace at which you run where you are at, or less than, 72% of your maximum heart rate. This is the ultimate zone as it allows for recovery and cardiovascular gains. There is an entire chapter on this later.

Phase Three (Speed Endurance)

Sunday	REST	Average resting HR: 48
Monday	28km run (24 x 800m at 3.45, 15 sec faster than goal race pace)	
Tuesday	10km run (zone 2)	
Wednesday	REST	
Thursday	28km run (15 x 1600m at 3.45, again 15 sec faster than race pace)	
Friday	10km run (Zone 2)	
Saturday	REST	
Sunday	6km run (Zone2)	Average resting HR: 46
Monday	21km run (6k, 5k ,4k, 3k, 2k, 1k with 90 sec rest, all at 15 sec faster than race pace), this was 2 km too far[24].	
Tuesday	Treatment	

---

[24] Schoolboy error as it resulted in a calf strain. I was therefore forced to take a week's rest from running. In that time, I remembered to be patient. Fitness is not lost if you are able to maintain blood flow to the muscles in the form of stretching. I was also needling myself every second day. Yes, with acupuncture needles. (More on this later.) This session was 2 km too far. This was my first marathon training attempt, so hopefully this lesson helps you.

Phase Four (Taper)

Wednesday	Treatment[25]	
Thursday	Treatment	
Friday	Treatment	
Saturday	Treatment	
Sunday	Treatment	
Monday	10km run (Zone 2)	Average resting HR: 43
Tuesday	REST	
Wednesday	10km run (Zone 2)	
Thursday	(Fly to New York)	
Friday	7km run (zone 2 with 10 x 30 sec at 3.45)	
Saturday	REST	
Sunday	RACE DAY	

---

[25] Trigger point needling, stretching, heat application, ice, strapping. At this point I was needling myself as I did not have the luxury of having a manual therapist work at my clinic every day. Looking back, it is extremely weird when you learn needling at university. You must needle yourself in 3rd year, for the first time, before you needle your classmates. The exact muscle you needle first is the muscle between your thumb and your index finger. You just stick it in there. *That's what she said.*

Seven-step Formula

Over this eight week period, I slept, on average, eight and a half hours per night. This meant sacrificing a few social invitations. It also meant prioritizing recovery.

I completely cut out alcohol from my diet for the five weeks before the race. Alcohol is a toxin to the body, therefore clean eating also means clean drinking, with lots of water and no artificial drinks. You will see later that my diet is primarily a hybrid of vegan and pescatarian. There is not much dairy or added sugar. Spoiler, there is a chapter dedicated to diet, particularly an anti-inflammatory diet.

Over the eight week preparation period, my average resting heart rate went from 52 to 43. This major drop signifies a major change in my running fitness and form and the turning point was the last of the 100km weeks.

Logically it made sense - this would be evidence of the body's adaption to the new training load. You will read later how recovery works and how the body undergoes supercompensation after physical stress. The body eventually becomes more efficient at supplying oxygen-rich blood to the muscles when they are pushed beyond limits that they have not exceeded before. In other words, your VO_2 max ("V" for volume, "O_2" for oxygen, and "max" for maximum) increases and your heart can pump more blood per beat, meaning that your heart rate goes down. This is rather important.

To summarize, here is my seven-step formula to your very own personal best race:

One: Be Consistent

The first and golden rule of training. Coach Clint[26] always stressed that. To be consistent, you need to avoid injury. To avoid injury, you need to be healthy. Fortunately, you have the blueprint on just how to do that in your hands (or your ears if you are listening to this) right now.

Two: Stay Healthy

Learn to listen to your body. The best way of doing this is using your heart rate, and more specifically, your resting heart rate. Prioritise your recovery. Recovery means getting enough sleep and eating clean. Staying physically healthy means monthly therapy sessions, at the least.

If you arrive at the race healthy, your body is designed to push into the red for many hours. If you arrive at a race healthy, you will also be able to recover quicker and recover fully afterwards.

This is the premise for how we can apply this recovery formula to health and wellness. Recovery, health, and fitness have to do with creating a healing environment within the body. And health and fitness are both directly proportional to the quality of your recovery. This is all explained very thoroughly in chapters to come.

---

[26] Clinton Gravett. Professional triathlete and professional friend. He is so liked that he is everybody's best man at their weddings. He taught me everything I know about training slower to become faster.

Three: Develop a *Huge* Muscle Memory Base

When you get tired, your muscles need to remember what they are supposed to do. The only way to do this is spend hours upon hours in Zone 2. This much slow running can be frustrating at times, but worth it.

I am certain you would have heard runners speaking about muscle memory. Well muscles do not have their own brains. Muscle memory is a nerve memory, that comes from your brain. To increase and improve your *muscle memory*, we focus on developing your Neural Re-Education. You do this with 90% of your running in Zone 2, 10% of your running in the Red Zone and by following a *Neural Re-Education* protocol[27].

Four: Cross Training

Cross training develops strength. Strength endurance is simply the ability to last longer at your desired speed. This is essential for the latter part of the marathon.

Cross training includes adding other types of exercise like cycling and swimming to your training regimen. Another form of strength endurance is body weight training. Body weight training includes core and proprioception, and any bodyweight functional exercises like burpees, squats and lunges.

It is not only about developing your cardiac and running efficiency, you also need an extremely functional muscular system. When your normal running muscles fatigue and you start to push yourself to maintain a good pace, your body will recruit other muscles to do so. The body is brilliant in that way. That is why you will see that runners at the end of the race will be running differently. It is their bodies becoming desperate to

---

[27] There will be forthcoming chapters on the two zones of training, Zone 2 and the Red Zone, and how these are related to health, fitness and recovery. Also, their relationship with Neural Re-Education, which is how we teach the brain what normal movement feels like again. It is a rather fascinating concept.

maintain the pace. As other muscles are recruited, their stride and their form alter slightly. It can sometimes not be pretty, and it can be almost agonising to watch.

Five: Run

Not only will you have to run, you will need some speed too. If you want to finish a marathon with a time that starts with "two hours", you are going to have to average 4.15min per km for the duration of the run. This is not as mind-blowing as Eliud's pace, or Nick's (you will meet him later), but it is still scary to think about.

If I had four months to train for a marathon, I would start to introduce 'Red Zone' sessions throughout my training weeks, but not too soon. To do this I would call Nick, ask him to coach me and join his *Track Tuesdays*. During the early stages of a marathon training block, start adding in noticeably short one-minute intervals at red zone intensity to help develop your running and cardiac efficiency[28]. This can also be improved by training with some form of resistance like running up hills.

Six: Quality over Quantity

That was how I was forced to do it with limited time. Looking back, that is how I will do it every time in the future, with maybe just a doubling of the program from an eight-week to a sixteen-week build-up.

If you choose to go out and simply smash loads of distance for the sake of it, that is okay, as long as you have the time and the body to handle it. Otherwise injury is inevitable for that

[28] Which I recommend. I will put this into practice for next year, 2021, hopefully at the Chicago Marathon!

mentality, unfortunately, and that breaks rule number one, being consistent. The main thing is to listen to your body. Learn to know when your body needs a Zone 2 recovery day, and when it is time to add Red Zone speed sessions, make them count.

Seven: Have Fun

Try not to take training and life too seriously. I promise you; you will have bad days and you will have bad sessions. I guarantee that you will most likely pick up a niggle or two along the way. Bad days and injuries are the result of our stressful and inflammatory-prone lifestyles. When the metaphorical pawpaw hits the fan, and all seems chaotic and lost, do not stress. Keep it simple and apply some of the principles in this book[29].

---

[29] In South Africa, instead of saying that the "sh*t has hit the fan", the less abrasive version is when "the *pawpaw hits the fan*". We call them Pawpaw's as South Africans (that is what my dad calls them) but we mean Papaya. Pawpaw's are small fruits, native to the United States and Canada and look quite different. Papaya are a large fruit that have a sweet soft orange flesh when they are ripe. They grow rampant in South Africa.

Race Report

The week before the race I spoke on the phone with Clint. We discussed the race strategy. The first option was to try and hold the 4.15 minutes per km needed to achieve 2:59, but this is risky as you have no wiggle room in case nature calls and you need to visit a Portapotty *en route*[30] or you cramp, or who knows, you may get tackled by someone in the crowd[31].

Also, there was the fact that I am a heavy runner, and it was my first marathon, meaning we did not know how my body would hold after 30km. I think Clint's exact words were *"you're going to die towards the end my friend"*. Forget the slowest possible way to die. This death would take only 3 hours if all went as planned. We agreed that if I felt good on race day, I would get as much of the distance out of the way as I could, without going into the red, and then rely on mental strength towards the end. In my head, I felt comfortable at four minutes per kilometre, and I therefore wanted to get 30km out of the way in two hours. This would give me one hour to run the remaining 12.2 km.

The New York marathon is unique in that it is the only one of the major marathons that does not start remotely near to the finish. This makes it a long day, as you need to leave four hours before the start time to get to Staten Island. At 5:00 a.m. we caught an Uber from the Upper East Side of Manhattan to the Whitehall Terminal on the south tip of the island. From here we caught a 5:30 a.m. ferry that takes you past the Statue of Liberty and drops you off on Staten Island. Then you join a

---

[30] This must be every runner's worst nightmare - having the need to do a number 2 during the race. I remember watching a certain professional female runner who did it in a live televised race (you can Google this), except she could not find a toilet in time. She just went on the road. I envy that. In Africa we love to do it outside. If you are surfing and you need to go, we call that a *H poo O*.

[31] These three are in decreasing risk of occurrence. Almost everyone will feel the need to go to the toilet during a marathon. Majority of runners will experience cramp in their legs. Getting tackled by someone in the crowd is an exceedingly rare occurrence.

queue to climb on a bus at around 6:30 a.m. that takes you to the start, arriving at Fort Wadsworth by 7:15 a.m. The wait in the Start Village is at least two hours, which is made easier with free food and thousands of nervous faces. This whole process brings a mixture of emotions. You are constantly thinking how astonishing it is to be there, whether or not you have trained enough, and if you will need to go to the toilet (before or during the race) or not. That last thought gives runners the most anxiety.

The gun went off and we were under way. The first two kilometres are uphill as you run over the Verrazzano-Narrows Bridge from Staten Island into Brooklyn. I felt good from the start. My first 10km were possibly too quick at 38.11, which translated into an average 3.49 minutes per km. Most of the first half of the marathon takes you through the streets of Brooklyn which are lined with cheering fans, live music bands and the smells of Brooklyn's diverse culinary delights. The halfway point (13 miles or 21 kilometres) is on the second of the bridge crossings, the Pulaski Bridge, which was our exit from Brooklyn and our entry into Queens. At the halfway mark I was 1.23.04, averaging 3.57 minutes per km.

During the next ten kilometres I could feel the fatigue starting to build up in my legs. Breathing becomes more laboured at this stage, and your body starts to feel a little less like your own. I noticed a wobble in what normally feels like a fluid running rhythm. We crossed the Queensboro Bridge into Manhattan for the first time and ran up First Avenue from 1st and 59th towards The Bronx. This was into the wind, which made it feel like running on a false flat.

At 30km, my time was 2.02.17 (an average of 4.03 per km). This was now officially the longest road run I had ever done. Clint's words were echoing in my mind now, "*you're going to die towards the end my friend"*, and I certainly was running out of steam. But this was the plan. We knew I wanted to get a big chunk of the distance under the belt, and I was only two minutes off my goal for 30km. Now was the time to dig deep.

If you ever do a marathon or even a half marathon, there comes a time when all you are doing in your head is one calculation after the next. You are constantly working out how far you have left, or if you have a time goal, how fast you need to be to cover the remaining distance. Fortunately, I have a good grasp of such sums, and I knew I needed to average a pace of 4.42 per km for the last twelve kilometres to get into the elusive 2% group.

My Garmin was on auto lap, meaning that after every kilometre it beeped and told me what my time was for the previous kilometre. Beep. 31st km, 4.20. Beep. 32nd km, 4.29. Beep. 33rd km, 4.31. I kept my focus on rhythm and breathing. I kept on reminding myself: *Keep your legs ticking over. Deep breaths.*

Beep. 34th km, 4.23. Even though this was a faster split, it was around this mark when negative thoughts started to enter my mind. It was approximately at the time we crossed the fourth bridge, the Willis Avenue Bridge, which you cross to enter The Bronx. You run two kilometres through The Bronx. You then enter Manhattan Island for the second and last time over the last of the bridges, the Madison Avenue Bridge.

The calculations in my head continued and I now knew I needed to average 4.45 per km for the last eight kilometres if I wanted to finish under three hours. By now, my body felt detached from myself, and I began to feel the desperation I mentioned earlier. My body was recruiting every muscle it could to propel me forward, including muscles I knew I had (from dissecting bodies), and from textbooks. But these were ones I had never felt before. I even developed a classic runners' headache (that dull thud behind your forehead.) This can only be explained by the muscles in and around your neck all starting to tighten up. Picture any grimacing runner you have seen on TV[32].

---

[32] There is a whole chapter later dedicated to common headaches. *More spoilers.*

Eight kilometres to go and I started talking to myself: *You have done hundreds, almost thousands, of 8km runs in your lifetime Cuan. Mostly with Kaylem. What is one more little run with your brother?*

Beep. 35th km, 4.36. I was hanging on. We were now running along Fifth Avenue. That road felt like it would never end. And to add insult, the elevation increases as you run up towards Central Park where the finish line is.

Then, almost instantly, came the lowest point of my race. There was a time during the 36th km that I thought to myself I would happily take a 3.05. That *this* is still *okay* for my first marathon. It is still a *good time*. I was physically hurting, and at times felt as though I was running backwards, a most bizarre sensation. For those few moments, which felt like a short stint in hell, I will admit that I had given up on my goal time. This kilometre was the one that emptied me of my motivation. I must have dropped to six minutes for this kilometre which would make it impossible to finish under three hours now.

I was beginning to accept that I had nothing left in the tank to push me onwards. Then, something happened. My Garmin beeped for the kilometre split time. I was expecting to see six something for the 36th km, as I was basically at a walking pace in my head. I looked at my watch and saw 4.36.

You have got this, Cuan. You have got this!

So many things went through my head at that moment. Just when I was looking for any motivation that might pull me out of the doldrums, I felt as though I had just been handed a 'get out of jail free' card. Even though it felt as though I was running backwards, that 36th km was still around ten seconds under the necessary pace to finish the race in less than three hours.

For the 37th km, the same thing happened, yet the time was 4.33, even though I still felt like I was fighting to keep an efficient rhythm. By now I started to think that I had some time to play with, which was needed, because the two kilometres up to and alongside Central Park was where the elevation increased even more.

I cannot perfectly recall these two kilometres. Within the blur of screaming fans and skyscrapers, the road began to climb. Everybody knows the feeling of trying to propel your bodyweight up a hill: It is simply impossible to keep the same pace as on a flat road. And all I focussed on here was getting one leg in front of the other one.

Beep. 38th km, 4.52. I had given some time back to the goal pace but considering the uphill I was content.

Beep. 39th km 4.53. I had given even more time back to the goal pace now. I really did not have any wiggle room.

The last five kilometres, from the 37th km onwards, is probably the part of the race where all you are thinking about is digging deep within yourself to get to the finish. This is when I reminded myself of the many times that I had *turned myself inside out* before. I thought back to races and runs where I had taught my body and mind to push on through the pain. I see many athletes calling this 'The Pain Cave' and that is rather accurate. I had flashbacks to my childhood and overcoming difficult times. As unpleasant as they are, these experiences grow you as a person and develop your self-confidence[33].

I suppose it is the last three kilometres that I shall remember most vividly. I entered Central Park, and all that lay between me and the finish line was a rolling road with a few uphill kinks.

The crowds throughout the entire race poured out encouraging cheers and applause, they almost lined the entire route – except for the bridges. The route in Central Park oozed a different level of crowd cheering energy. I knew I just needed to keep my legs moving and I should reach my 'Sub-

---

[33] Another spoiler for later but self-confidence for me goes hand in hand with my spirituality. The power of the human spirit (aka digging deep) is such a privilege, provided that you are *able* to move. It comes from a place of humility as some people are confined to wheelchairs and physically cannot move.

3' time goal. But I was hurting. Hurting badly.

Beep. 40th km, 4.36. I was back on track. I remember being caught up in deafening drumming, electric guitars, and ringing bells. And the smell of doughnuts from a food truck. If ever there was a scene set for a movie finish, it was now; it was time to leave it all on the road.

Beep. 41st km, 4.33. As you run through this famous setting, you remember happy scenes from movies like *Breakfast at Tiffany's* and *Big Daddy*. You remember the smiles on the faces of your family back home. You remember what a privilege it is to travel, to have an able body, to be able to feel pain. Some people cannot. You remember the reasons you wanted to do this in the first place. The mind goes where it needs to, to not think about the body's near shutdown.

Beep. 42nd km, 4.16. This was quick. I always back my finishing kick. There is always more than you think left in the tank.

There was now 200m left, and it was about 15m before the finish line that a litre of green Gatorade energy drink hurtled out of my mouth. I have thrown up a few times in my life, but this was by far the most pleasurable. Warm and green, like a humid summer's day, I never even flinched. I wiped my mouth, and my body dropped over the line[34].

2.59.07.

Never in my wildest dreams could I have scripted the race better. After any big run, you almost need to remind your body how to walk again. Once I could, I began the long walk back to where our supporters were waiting with food at the entrance

---

[34] Let me explain why you throw up during exercise. It can be linked to dehydration (sweating too much and losing electrolytes) and voluntarily drinking too many fluids in the race that do not have enough electrolytes in them to replace the lost electrolytes. To avoid dehydration; therefore, your body throws it up. Or imagine that all your blood is getting sent to your legs and arms to keep you moving. Your organs now do not have enough blood supply and before they collapse, they too will throw up their contents. Throwing up is welcomed by some runners who cannot hold their bowel contents.

to Central Park. I had a real sense of gratitude and a smile that almost caused my cheeks to cramp. And what a treat that would have been - the first cramps of the day.

Until my next marathon, *Deo volente*, in Chicago. And a challenge of 2.55.

It was during my flight back to London the next evening that I had this epiphany. I remember the moment clearly because my body was so sore that standing up and going to the toilet was a victory in itself. I sat there and reflected on how I had reached this milestone in my life. I reflected on what factors had contributed to this major personal victory.

Then I realised that I had already started writing a book, which happens to be about these exact topics - diet, pain, headaches, recovery, exercise, NRE, optimism, training schedules etc. It was at that moment that I knew I had an opportunity to share my life's journey to date. To share my formula for a healthy life. The Marathon was the motivation I needed to finish this book.

Challenge accepted.

Point to ponder: The power of the mind is astronomically greater than you think, do not doubt that you have this genius inside of you.

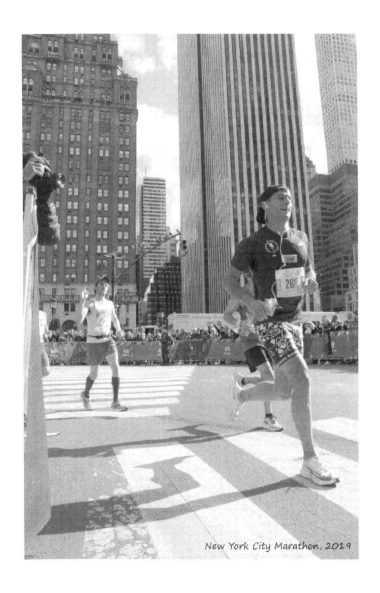

New York City Marathon, 2019

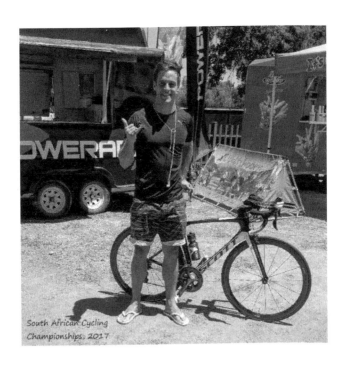

South African Cycling
Championships, 2017

3 : Moving South Africa

Jon also describes a history of left medial knee pain while running. 7-year onset. Occasional monthly locking sensation that patient has to "wiggle" out of place. Pain usually starts after 8-10km of running. Jon says his knee feels "unstable" at times. *Pretty obvious what is wrong.*

My life to date can be reduced to two words: *movement* and *medicine.* Any reference to movement implies moving the way you were designed to move. Freely. Any reference to medicine is not to medication or drugs, rather it is a reference to health care. And by health care I mean creating an internal healing environment. More on these later. For now, just know that both are a privilege.

This stage of learning is called: Growing up.

The next two chapters are full of anecdotal stories,

memories or experiences that do not necessarily link up. These stories have moulded me into who I am today and have impacted my realisation of why movement is medicine. Their purpose serves as the multifaceted background to how movement has transformed my life in one way or another. Hopefully after these two chapters you know a little more about *why* I do what I do.

Let us start in South Africa.

Durban

I was born in Durban, in the eighties. But only just. It was in fact in 1989. This was a generation known for moustaches and mullets, but also a generation that played in sand and not on mobile phones. Life seemed uncomplicated and was spent primarily outside. The first personal computer was released only in the early eighties and this began the fall of movement as we know it. Even the Berlin Wall moved in 1989, which for a wall, is quite something.

I am eternally grateful for my parents and the upbringing they offered me. We grew up with everything we needed, not everything that we wanted.

The friend that I have known the longest is Jabin[35]. We grew up together in Durban. Our parents were friends and that was how we became friends. We were born six months apart and we did everything together. Some of our fondest memories were exploring the quiet streets of Gillitts (a suburb in the hills of Durban where we both lived) on our bicycles. This was followed by numerous types of ball games in our backyard until it got too dark to safely continue. Eventually we would succumb to our mother's requests to come back inside the

---

[35] Jabin Lyons. Entrepreneur, freelance pastor, passionate friend and brand developer. Reminds me constantly of what is important in life. Makes me question my motive for doing things. That trait I believe is gold in the 21st century.

house. We have one printed photograph from 1993 of the two of us on these tiny plastic motorbikes, the ones we used when we were about four years old.

Movement meant freedom from your parents; movement was life at the time.

Johannesburg

My family then moved to Johannesburg when my father was reassigned there for work. My father worked for Transnet; a transport company with a skeleton of infrastructure throughout the country to move goods around. Johannesburg (Joburg or Jozi as it is called by the locals) is where I, at the age of six, started primary school. It is a concrete jungle. Known also as eGoli, the *City of Gold*, as it was built on mining and the industries that fed off it[36].

Ever since I can remember I have had a stutter. Thirty years down the line it may be a well-hidden one, but it is still *there*. It was burdensome when I was a child, as other children love to tease anything, or anyone, who they perceived as *abnormal*. Should my stammer be the closest I ever get to a disability, I would consider myself incredibly lucky. I am also grateful that it has given me an appreciation for being different. Being unique is not a choice. We are all unique in some way, even though I do feel sometimes that society as a whole is becoming more robotic. But as with all hardships, especially in our younger years, I believe God knows what we can handle. I developed a coping mechanism called 'competitiveness'; and the drive and determination to win, and so prove the denigrators wrong. I did this not out of hate, but out of love for

---

[36] Even so, it was here that my passion for sport was sparked as a young boy. We played soccer, or football as it is known on in the UK. My brother and I soon became involved in running and in a sport called biathlon, which is basically triathlon without the bicycle.

who God made me to be. Over the years I have learnt not to shy away from a challenge, instead I am thrilled when I am challenged, particularly in public speaking[37].

Movement meant competitiveness; movement was learning new skills.

The Moon

Medically, this is how a stutter works. Parts of the lower right section of your brain are particularly active when speech movements stop. Now if this region is overactive, it hinders other brain areas that are involved in the starting and ending of speech movements. It is as simple as that.

A stutter is weird, and it is difficult to explain what takes place in my mind when it happens. Let me try. Take any sentence I am thinking about verbalising. As I am speaking, I can foresee the words I want to use, and I know which words are potentially hazardous. So, before I get there, I search for a different word, (if I know one), or I throw in an 'um' and that often allows me to avoid stumbling on a word. You may notice a few 'um's if you watch any of the YouTube videos on which I feature. Now you know what those 'ums' signify. They are "avoidance strategies", and they are like superpowers.

Here is an example of that superpower when it was not yet fully harnessed. Let me paint the picture. I was eight years old. We were living in Johannesburg where frost is common in winter. One morning I went outside and our wooden decking outside was frozen over.

Naturally, I saw this as an opportunity to attempt to moonwalk as I had seen Michael Jackson do so many times. I reckon, with the aid of slippery ice, I absolutely nailed it. Ecstatic at my potential dancing future, I needed to tell

---

[37] Even to this day, hearing me speak on a stage is like watching a dog walk upright on its back legs. Even if it is not done well, you are amazed it can be done at all.

someone, so I sprinted into my parents' bedroom and as quickly and excitably as possible shouted out 'Dad, Mom, I did a mmmmmmmmm. Mmmmmmmmm. Mmmmm[38]. By the fourth second of constant humming, I eventually get out the rest of the word "moonwalk". My parents laughed, not at me, but at the *cuteness* of it. I joined the laughter, but at the same time was acutely aware of how silly I sounded when I tried to get certain words out and found myself stuck on the first letter. I never thought it was cute. When I look back, I can appreciate the inherent innocence and vulnerability of such a childhood experience, it is a story that I can now laugh about at family reunions, but at the time feeling different and silly was something I had to digest.

Later, in my primary school years, speech therapy would prove to be a great help. The therapist would advise me to take a deep breath before problematic words. The therapists would draw a molehill, whilst I was, symbolically at least, an ant. The ant climbs up the hill, which represents inhaling. As the ant descends the molehill, which represents breathing out, I would then exhale the word I wanted to say. Deep breath. "Moonwalk" as I breathe out. In my mind it made sense for some reason or another, a rhythmic breath outwards almost forces the word out. I embraced the technique, and used it when tricky words cropped up, but it took me years before I could notice a marked improvement from practising this technique. What it taught me, however, was that movement was needed to become an efficient speaker.

Movement here meant speech; movement meant conversation.

---

[38] It was normally on the third audible mmmmmm that I started swearing in my head. It was very frustrating growing up. It still is today.

The Farm

Every year, while we were living in Johannesburg, we would visit our grandparents at the coast. My mother's parents were farmers in Brakfontein, just outside of the city of East London. My brother and I agree that these were some of the most enjoyable times of our lives. The thing about these holidays is that we never stopped moving.

One of the fondest memories we have was of something that happened on the farm. My grandad Mic had a small vegetable and dairy farm. We would run and play our hearts out. We would shoot as many birds[39] as we could with pellet guns. The understanding that underpinned the bird-shooting was that we had to eat what we killed. We would build fires made from wood we collected around the farmland and cook the birds on the braai[40]. My dad taught Kaylem and me how to initially de-feather and gut the birds. Once we were confident, we could do it on our own. All the birds we shot were edible. They tasted like sweet chicken mixed with whatever spice my gran gave us. The children of the staff on the farm would always join us. By now, they were our best friends.

There were numerous families who worked and lived on the farm. Many of them lived in hand-built huts. We would often play soccer with the children of the staff members until it was dark. For some kids and grandkids of farmers like my grandad Mic, this was perhaps normal or acceptable, but for many other South Africans who had become accustomed to the normality of segregated races under Apartheid, it would have been considered absurd. But this was six years post-

---

[39] The common birds that we were allowed to shoot, with Pappa Mic's permission, were finches. More specifically the cuckoo-finch, also known as a parasitic weaver. They ate the chicken's feed. They would sit on the fence of the chicken coop by the hundreds.

[40] A braai is the South African term for a wood fire or coal barbeque. A gas barbeque is not a real barbeque according to most South Africans.

apartheid, and for us kids, all we cared about was having fun together, regardless of race or any other categories of difference that society deemed important. Plastic crates were used as goalposts, and we played on a field that had more holes than a dartboard. Sometimes we would visit the farm in Winter, and the same rules and routines applied, with one important difference. Our feet would freeze on the winter grass, and the only remedy was to jump feet first into a fresh heap of steaming cow dung. The warmth would slither between our toes and engulf our feet. When you cannot feel your feet from the cold, this was almost revitalizing.

My granddad taught us to wake up early. Cows needed to be milked, and we would roll out of bed at 04:30 to help and be back for breakfast at 6:00. We would drink milk; full cream, unpasteurized, straight from the udder, with all the bad stuff[41].

Once the cattle were milked, the milk needed to be sold. We would drive with Grandad Mic through the rural post-apartheid townships selling fresh milk for R1.00 a litre, (that's 5p in British terms). As young boys we would be on the back of the *bakkie* (South African pickup truck) shouting out in isiXhosa *"nanku amasi, nanku amas-ey"*. Which, in the rural townships at the time, meant *here is the milk. Here is the milk[42]*.

---

[41] Refer to the *Clean Eating* chapter, but in my opinion, the only form of dairy that we should have is the unpasteurized milk from free range animals such as the ones on my grandad's farm. These bacteria are great for your gut health. Louis Pasteur's pasteurization process, of course, is essential to kill harmful organisms, especially ones found in the 21st century dairy process.

[42] Amasi refers to sour or fermented milk in Xhosa. Ubisi is the correct Xhosa word for the milk we were selling. Linguistically it may not make sense in English, but the way the Xhosa language communicates is different. Words communicate meaning in a more abstract or creative way than in English, in this case words that make the melody sound better.

We would shout that from the bottom of our developing lungs, as loudly as we could[43].

Movement was realizing our privilege; movement was gratitude.

East London

Then came my high school years. We moved from *Joburg* when I was twelve years old. My brother and I went to school in East London, a city on the East Coast of South Africa. Selborne College, the high school I attended, is an all-boys school. It is based on manly traditions[44]. If you played in the first rugby team, you were a walking god in the school community. My brother and I were runners, scrawny, and we did not play rugby. We were therefore not gods. There is a fortunate upside to this: we may have healthy joints in our old age. Let us wait and see. You would imagine that sport was the focus over academics at a boys' school, and you would be right, although academics were always verbally prioritised. My brother and I were somewhat nerds. The kind of nerds who also participated in sport. What we both learnt quickly was that our sporting ability seemed to benefit our academic results and earn us a few 'get out of jail free' cards. Our running coach was also our geography teacher. Sometimes it felt like even multiple-choice answers were marked in our favour.

In his final year of secondary school, my bother Kaylem was Selborne's golden boy, the Head boy of the school and the top performing academic. Walking out of a geography exam

---

[43] From these kinds of memories, we learnt the basic life lesson that happiness is often found in simplicity. As kids, my brother and I grew up with everything that we needed; not everything that we wanted. Appreciation became a way of life. I will forever be grateful for that.

[44] It is a school that I am proud to say I attended. Selborne College celebrated respect, love, manners, loyalty, a strong work ethic, and unity.

he boldly claimed that the answer to question number 2B was a "warm" front, when it was most certainly a "cold" front. His friends laughed at him as he had finally got something incorrect. At that moment, a teacher walked past, and was asked what the correct answer was. Obviously, a "cold" front. Everyone erupted with laughter again and explained that Kaylem had finally got one answer wrong. The teacher immediately offered an explanation along the likes of 'well you see gentleman; it could be a warm front as a warm front always precedes a cold front.' This was a classic case of being handed a 'get out of jail free' card.

Kaylem, who is two years older than I am, became a world champion in biathle, at the World Championships in Germany in 2005. He then went on to study medicine. I always knew I would apply for medicine or chiropractic when I completed my schooling. My first World Championship Competition for biathle was the year after, which also happened to be my first overseas trip. It took place in Monaco. Monaco, I quickly learned was the James Bond of travels, where yachts and sportscars were the norm. I managed a fourth place (the first of the real losers to be out of the medals) but still, what a trip to open my eyes to the big world. There were all those opportunities. Sport opened almost as many doors as good manners did.

Movement was opportunity; movement meant travel.

Johns Hopkins University

While I biatheled in Monaco, my good friend Brett made the national squash team. We played field hockey together, both on the left-hand side of the field. We had similar academic interests, and both loved a good competition. Academically, Brett is the cleverest person I know[45], and like

---

[45] Brett would probably correct that to 'most clever', but it is my book after all.

my brother he was the top performing academic at our school. He taught me the words "indefatigable" and "incandescence" - when he was just sixteen! Our sporting achievements bolstered our applications for the People to People Future Leaders Summit, and we were selected to attend in the USA. We both experienced our first taste of College life. My particular summit was on medicine, for potential future medical doctors, at Johns Hopkins University. We were accommodated in university dormitories and ate real fast food. But the lessons we learnt there still shape us to this day. It was there, at Johns Hopkins University, that I learnt that prevention truly is better than cure. It was thirteen years ago, but I remember the words I heard there. *"The only way to cure a gunshot DOA (dead on arrival) is to prevent it."*

Movement meant exposure to the big wide world; movement became a vision of preventative medicine.

Dad and Mom

I know playing sport is not everyone's cup of tea. For my brother and me it was something we felt naturally drawn to. Perhaps it was knitted into our DNA from conception. My father Wayne[46] played semi-professional rugby and my mother Bridgette[47] was a track and field sprinter, who held local records for many years. Sport and exercise were always a major part of our lives and my brother and I fared well in track, triathlon, duathlon and lifesaving. Yes, lifesaving is a

---

[46] Wayne Coetzee. Father, provider and master of dad-humour. He taught me that if you want something, you need to work hard for it. Life does not give out freebies. An example of a true giver, which is probably where I get it from.

[47] Bridgette Coetzee. Beautiful. Mother, comforter and textbook overthinker. I am a mommy's boy, a title I am grateful for as the reality is that many people do not have a mom. Just as you thought this book was only about movement and me trying to be funny.

sport. I am not currently, by profession, a saver of lives *per se*, but indirectly I would accept that description of my work if one considers that the pursuit of health can add years on to one's life. Every single day, to this day, I try and do some form of exercise, even if it is just a stretch or a ten minute core session. It is never too late in the day, or in one's life, to exercise, and the session can never be too short.

My mother's dream was to be a doctor. She is brilliant and had a passion for health as a young woman. However, as owners of a small farm in South Africa, there was no money to send her to study. Maybe it was this passion that rubbed off onto my brother and me. My brother, as you know, is now a medical doctor and specialist orthopaedic surgeon[48]. He, too, is one of the smartest people I know.

Another case.

February 2005

Jesse Pinkman, a 16-year-old schoolboy presented to the clinic. He is a smart, happy-go-lucky student with aspirations of becoming a cook one day.

Patient presents with a sub-acute low back pain following an incident where he was hit by a car whilst cycling. Arachnoiditis is ruled out[49].

X-rays were justified and taken, primarily to further rule out possible spinal stress fractures.

He is diagnosed with multiple facet joint strains in the

---

[48] You may have noticed I do love to speak highly of my brother and how exceptional the guy is at life. I cannot help being proud of him. Even when at university he thought that "double spacing" was hitting the "space bar" on the keyboard twice between every word. True story.

[49] This is inflammation of the arachnoid, which is the middle layer of the spinal canal covering. This covering is like a pipe that encompasses the spinal cord, nerve roots, (known as the cauda equina), and protective fluid that flows inside the canal.

lumbar and thoracic spine and Jesse responded to chiropractic mobilizations.

The good-to-knows:

ONE. The pain was affecting his training and hence his chances of racing national triathlon champs the following month.

TWO. Pain medication was not helping, which was the reason for the consultation.

THREE. Restoring movement was the main mechanism of healing and he made the national triathlon team two weeks later.

Movement meant returning to sport; movement becomes my job.

Durban (Round Two)

Before I forget, let me make this extremely clear: please regard any reference to medicine or doctors in this book as a friendly dig at my brother - someone who always challenges my advice or suggestions.

After school I went to study Chiropractic in Durban at the age of eighteen. If you were counting, I had by now spent six years in each of Durban, *Joburg*, East London and was now set on another six in Durban. This number keeps following me.

We have been taught so much more about shame than we have about our own anatomy. I discovered that Anatomy is also much more fun when studied in a private, co-educational environment.

Something you do not expect from a chiropractic degree is that we study anatomy in the same way a surgeon would, and we do anatomical dissections, on real cadavers, for two years. Yes, we were each given a body which we slowly dismantled for two years. All the sweetcorn, (that is what fat looks like between your fingers), and any other tissue removed from the body went into a bin next to our dissection tables, and after two years that bin and what was left of the body were cremated[50].

When I look back now, I realise that dissection is invaluable. It sets you apart from degrees that do not include dissections. When I stick a needle into your upper trapezius at the base of your neck, which is awfully close to your lungs, I do so with confidence because I know exactly how deep to go. This is because I have cut a trapezius muscle in every direction that it can be cut.

I lived in the hostel or residence (cost effective student housing) and as it goes the food is inadequate for a growing young man. I was always hungry. Dissection days were not everyone's favourite. For a few reasons. This was mainly because you smelled like death for the whole day. By death I mean you smelled like the preservative chemical formaldehyde, which allows you to keep a body for two years. The smell of formaldehyde sticks to your hands and it cannot be easily washed off. The odour lingers in your sinuses and you smell death all day. One lunch break after dissections, Peta's mother had made her a pork sandwich. If you did not know, human meat is identical to pig meat, and as Peta put the sandwich to her mouth, she saw death and smelt it on her fingers. She nearly gagged. I was there to rescue the sandwich for human consumption, and I promptly obliged by doing the honours. I know we were surrounded by dead bodies, but it looked as if Peta had seen a ghost. The medical emergency students (studying to become paramedics) would use our cadavers in their anatomy course. We would often move the organs around to try and trick them. Imagine opening the chest cavity and the first thing you see is a heap of small intestines. In hindsight this was not smart. These are the people we need to save our lives.

---

[50] I have already signed up to donate my body to science when I die. I recommend it. It is not as glorious as what Will Smith did in SEVEN POUNDS, but it will change someone's life.

Movement here was satisfying hunger.

You quickly learn that the human body is very resilient. In my first year at university I was still competitive in duathlon and the week leading up to the national championships I was reminded of that. Whilst I was cycling in the cycling lane in central Durban, I was not concentrating. Perhaps as a result of sheer fatigue, I lost focus and allowed my front wheel to make contact with the wheel of my training buddy. Luckily, I fell onto my left shoulder and was wearing a helmet, which shattered on the tar. However, with the fall on my left, the bicycle fell towards the right and into the vehicle lane next to us, just as a large carrier truck was driving passed. The driver was in his lane and did nothing wrong. The bicycle went under the wheels and was pushed up and mangled into pieces. Fortunately, other than severe roasties (the speed at which you hit the tar produces such a friction force that your skin roasts as it is being scraped), I was mostly fine. We helped the truck driver get the remnants of the bicycle out from inside his wheel arch. He said that he saw me fall and he thought that the bump he felt under his truck was my body.

You never know what is around the next corner. Movement reminds you that life is fleeting.

New Zealand

For my 21st birthday present, my parents gave me a choice of gifts. I could choose between a party for all my friends or an overseas return flight. The choice was between gaining street credibility from my friends for some free alcohol, or a new life experience. *Is the Pope Catholic?* There was no choice in it. The real choice was: *where do I go?* Try deciding for yourself, if you were offered tickets right now, where you would go? For some, it is an easy answer to a lifelong dream to travel somewhere. Hawaii. Tokyo. Maldives.

After I investigated the status of my bank account as a

student, my decision was circumscribed by the availability of charity-priced accommodation. Now the list was down to what family and friends we had overseas. One of Nicole's (then my brother's girlfriend[51]) friends had recently moved to New Zealand with her family, and Nicole had been promising to visit her. Nicole, Kaylem and I decided to go to the land of the long white cloud, *Aotearoa*, to try find Bilbo Baggins in the Shire.

Besides this being one of the most beautiful scenic countries on the planet, where we ran trails alongside glaciers and speed-boated next to cliffs, it was during this trip that my brother hurt himself. Or so we thought. Towards the end of the trip he developed a shooting and excruciating pain, starting in his lower back and extending down his leg. It was accompanied by fever and chills and was the worst physical pain he had felt to date. We have had many brotherly fights and physical encounters and I can see when Kaylem is genuinely in pain. He was not joking - this pain was defeating him.

At the time I had just finished my third year of chiropractic studies, so I was a self-proclaimed adjuster[52]. Kaylem had just completed 5th year at medical school at the University of Cape Town. This gave him, (and me), limited medical legitimacy credentials, and together we self-diagnosed him as having a disc injury. *It had to be.*

Without a budget for treatment abroad, the only thing we could think of was to let me adjust him. So, I lay him down, rotated his leg over his body, lined up an L5/S1 adjustment,

---

[51] Nicole Coetzee. Now married to my brother, incredible mother, loving wife and sister. Mother to my hero, Cammy, and my other hero, Scott. That makes her my hero too.

[52] Chiropractic adjustment. The clicking thing. It helps restore movement and can help reduce your pain. Hopefully at the end of this book you will see how this may play a role in your road to regaining movement. How it plays a role in *Neural Re-education.*

and "Whack!" His back released amazingly. (*Release* is a term we use in chiropractic.) It is when you can clearly feel or hear a joint move, and if it was a joint that was restricted, you will often hear a cracking sound. (More on crack later- the chiropractic kind.)

Kaylem was free of pain for the next few hours (refer to the *Pain* chapter to understand how pain relief is obtained). As you can imagine, this 21-year-old chiropractic student was peacocking around claiming how great I was, and how good the adjustment had been. Kaylem even gave a nod of approval.

However, the pain soon came back - and with a vengeance. Now we had two days left and my brother was really battling. Pain intensity was increasing and accompanied by fever, and chills. Kaylem was confined to bed. He could not bear any weight on his leg. Red flags.

We had not told my parents yet. They are real worry pots when it comes to their sons, but before we boarded the flight home, I needed to tell them. This is how the phone call went.

Hi Mom and Dad. So, we are all good, leaving New Zealand now. See you in Cape Town. By the way, Kaylem will be getting off the plane in a wheelchair. Okay, love you. Bye.

If you can add some dramatic flair to life, why not?

Our flights went via Singapore, so Nicole and I went on our own adventures as Kaylem was literally man down. We landed in Cape Town the following day and boarded an ambulance straight to Groote Schuur Hospital, where Kaylem was admitted and the first MRI was done. For his back, as *it had to be* a disc, right? Third and fifth year student diagnoses. Then the MRI report of his lower back came back.

NAD[53].

---

[53] No Abnormality Detected. To cover yourself legally, you need always to document everything you do and say to a patient. To a student, NAD covered it all. It is like the "Please Call Me" text message service with the words "it's over", encompassing an entire breakup conversation.

Except for a small area of white in the hip musculature. You will see an example of this later, but depending on the contrast used, white on MRI often means fluid. *White* in real life sometimes means *privilege*.

Doctors then conducted an MRI of his hip and femur. This result was not NAD. Massive fluid build-up in the femur, sinus formation and exudate into the quadriceps muscle were detected. He had an osteomyelitis. This is a rare condition.

Now infections are easy to treat when you know the cause. Virus. Bacteria. Fungal. Except that, Kaylem's blood tests came back as NAD. That meant *nothing* was causing this infection. Red flag. Symptoms that cannot be attributed to a cause are obviously almost impossible to treat. Similarly, in my chiropractic's, if you cannot identify the root cause by reproducing the pain or have a patient responding to a short course of conservative treatment based on the likely differential diagnosis, this is a red flag.

When this happens in hospitals, doctors will throw the whole textbook at the patient (not literally), including broad spectrum antibiotics, anti-viral, and antifungals. In the meantime, they will try to grow a culture of the infection in a laboratory and attempt to identify it from there.

This took six weeks. In that time Kaylem needed to have surgery to decompress the bone pressure. Pain from internal bone pressure is clinically the worst. My apologies to any mother who has given birth naturally, please direct your hate towards the literature (which may be biased and which was probably written by a group of European men many years ago who perhaps did not think much of childbirth and often wondered why women were 'making such a fuss' during labour).

Eventually the doctors identified what was causing the infection, a fusobacterium. This is *extremely* rare. The antidote was given and Kaylem's prognosis went from "*remove the* leg" to *"you'll probably run again".*

When rare things happen, doctors put them into journals. Here is an extract from the South African Journal of Surgery:

An unusual case of an immunocompetent young adult with osteomyelitis and pyomyositis of his right thigh is presented. Despite the absence of typical clinical signs, a high index of suspicion and 16S RNA PCR led to an early diagnosis of Fusobacterium infection and subsequent successful multidisciplinary treatment.

Besides the variable clinical features of Fusobacterium infection, other factors can cause delay in diagnosis and therefore appropriate treatment. Firstly, human Fusobacterium infection is extremely rare, and most specialists will not see it during their medical career. Secondly, the metastatic manifestations can lead to erroneous diagnoses and in that regard cause initial presentation to a wide variety of specialties. Thirdly, as with many other anaerobic organisms, identification of Fusobacterium can be complicated and time consuming.

As you will see later, another member of our family also makes an appearance in a medical journal.

Years of re-x-rays of his leg eventually support the claim that it is in full remission - an answer to prayer. Also, the fact is that it never changed his sporting capabilities, and since then he has run circles around me on numerous occasions.

When rare and bad things happen, we can blame the world, we can blame someone, we can blame ourselves, many people blame God, some of us become angry, some of us give up there and then, and some of us use it as a crutch. Kaylem took a different approach and tried to see how he could benefit others from this experience. As an orthopaedic surgeon, he most certainly will have cases of osteomyelitis to deal with. You can bet your money that he will know what to do when they present, but also, he will have compassion and sympathy for

the patient and family, and that is what makes a real doctor[54].
Movement meant remission; movement was life or death.

Mordor

During this New Zealand trip, one of the tourist things we did was *the big night*, which was a deal in Queenstown that incorporated six pubs, a guide for the night and a group of students. The deal included an alcoholic beverage at each stop.

We were told that the night would end at the sixth pub at which there would be a special competition with a secret prize for the winner. We got to the last destination with slowed reflexes. That is what we told our parents. We were actually just tipsy. Now we got to the competition which on that night was a classic limbo, "how low can you go?". *Confident Cu* ended up winning, and I won a ticket to do the biggest bungie swing in the world the next day. It was an added treat that the next day I was not hanging like a painting and I experienced my first free fall experience at the Nevis Arch which was a suspended swing in the mountains of Mordor. Truly, that is where they filmed parts of the Lord of the Rings.

Movement meant free stuff. Movement was opportunity.

---

[54] It helps having a doctor in the family. Free scripts. But also: Once, on a hunt, my dad fell into a ditch and landed square on his thigh. The pain was so bad that at the time he said it must have been broken. Now a broken femur is no joke as you can bleed out if it nicks your femoral artery. Kaylem checked his femoral pulse and the whole hunt ended abruptly. We splinted his leg and we rushed him to the emergency room. The three of us are sitting on the back of the pickup, along with two animal carcasses that are leaking blood. We arrive at the ER entrance, and the scene must have looked like a chainsaw massacre. After opening the back of the pickup truck and blood poured out. It turns out, my dad only had a dead leg. He will now officially never live this down. The makeshift splint we used is in his bar room to this day.

Johannesburg (Round Two)

We start treating patients in our fifth year of studies[55]. I decided I needed to have an option to legally treat patients in a gym without doing a one- to three-year personal training course. I always wanted to do something that gave me permission to be in the gym, not that I felt I needed it, but you are still wet behind the ears when you are 23 years old. I researched many options, and one of them was a CrossFit coaches' course.

A few weeks later, and after minimal studying, I went to Johannesburg and attended *CrossFit Jozi* to complete the course. I was extremely fit at the time, both cardiovascularly from triathlon and strength wise, from gym work. I was also extremely confident[56].

The course was designed around the CrossFit method. CrossFit is a strength and conditioning program consisting mainly of a mix of aerobic exercises, calisthenics, and Olympic weightlifting. CrossFit as a brand describes its strength and conditioning program as "constantly varied functional movements". The course was three days long. It was mostly theoretical work, with practical portions where we were able to coach each other on the correct movement standards we had learnt that day. The main lesson I take from the course is that the manner in which your body can learn a neuromuscular firing pattern as a child, you will never lose as an adult.

---

[55] Working at a chiropractic clinic can be tricky sometimes because you can seldomly call in sick. Me: "Yeah, so, I can't come in today, my back hurts." Clinic director: "Come on in, we'll check you out."

[56] Before we continue: How do you know that someone does CrossFit? They will tell you. The same joke applies to vegans.

Let me explain. We all lose our basic flexibility because we move from playgrounds to school desks (if you are fortunate enough to go to school), roughly at the age of six. We lose our basic abdominal core activation as we rely more on backrests from chairs and vehicle seats, again roughly age six. The opposite side of the spectrum is that children who continue with gymnastics and extra-functional movement regimes after the age of six will never lose that firing pattern.

The exercise that we all had to attempt during the course was a "ring muscle up". Imagine you are hanging suspended in the air by your arms between two hanging gymnastics rings. The muscle-up begins with your arms extended above the head, gripping a hold in the rings. Your body is then explosively pulled up by your arms, with much greater speed than a regular pull-up. When your hands approach your upper chest, your body is leaned forward, and your elbows are straightened by activating your triceps. The routine is considered complete when the rings are at the level of your waist and your arms are fully straight. You are holding yourself between the rings. It sounds easy, please try it.

Because it is an advanced exercise, muscle-ups are typically first learned with an assistive kip, which is an aggressive leg swing up to provide momentum and to assist in the explosive upward force needed to ascend above the rings. My attempt at the ring muscle up must have looked ridiculous. I was doing a full body kip to try propelling myself above the rings, and I admit - I could not do it. Everybody tried, and almost everybody failed.

Someone in the group was a 45-year-old gentleman. He mentioned that he had done gymnastics as a young child. He stood back and watched all of us youngsters fail with horrendous form. We all assumed that the day was over when we all failed. Until Mr Miyagi got up and asked if he could have a go. I laughed on the inside, and I know others were too as some of them were laughing out loud. Then Miyagi jumped into the rings, and with pure elegance, pulled himself upwards, slowly, I had never seen anything so controlled before, no swing or kip needed, and his arms moved forward as he pushed himself into the air. The whole box went silent. It was as quiet as a catholic church in there. It was in that moment that I realised the importance of bringing up children with a *movement mindset*. Over the next few months, I practised technique, and as young Ralf Macchio, (the original Karate Kid) did, I was finally able to perform a half decent ring muscle up. And in that moment, I realised that it is never too late to teach the body how to move.

Movement was muscle memory; movement meant respect your elders.

Durban University of Technology

My fourth year at university was the year I met Luke[57]. He was also from East London and had just moved to Durban to also study chiropractic. We ended up living together in my final and sixth year. And we both ended up in London together. We had some great memories from university. A fond memory from our Durban days was during Tropical Storm Irina. She brought 15-foot waves to Durban's coastline which closed the beaches. Nevertheless, we decided to seize the opportunity, and grabbed our swimming flippers to swim out and body surf these waves. Luke was knocking on the Olympic swimming team's door and even he battled to get to the backline. As a wave broke in front of us, we would have to take a big breath and dive under the surging turbulent water. This would smash our bodies against the sandy seabed. The pressure of the water would force us against the ocean floor

---

[57] Dr Luke Pendock. Compassionate chiropractor, future successful businessman and great friend. He almost qualified to swim in the Olympic Games. We have a current and ongoing 9-year long argument whether Tiger Woods' eye laser enhancement surgery benefitted his golf game. You tell me?

for up to fifteen seconds, after which we would resurface behind the broken wave and swim as many strokes as possible towards the backline until the next wave broke. This continued for around twenty minutes until we eventually got to the backline. The backline is where the swell is, the waves are not breaking here. Absolutely exhausted, Luke and I just floated in the water, in the pouring rain, overlooking the craziness of Durban's city centre. There was a deafening silence as these swells passed underneath us. These six-meter swells, the size of a single-story house, passed under us with dreadful power yet with delicate serenity. We just floated there and basked in nature as she showed off her strength.

During the six years I spent at university, I was only almost kicked out twice. The second time was not my fault. We were in our fifth year, in a paediatric chiropractic lecture, and our lecturer told us that she had been in labour for more than twenty-four hours. In my somewhat childish mind, that was the equivalent of doing involuntary abdominal crunches for more than a day. In the gym world that equates to a six pack. I did not realise that natural birth often tends to rip the vaginal canal, as part of the normal birthing process. Now with six pack abdominals in my head, I put up my hand to highlight a potentially positive aspect of this lengthy labour and asked her if afterwards she was *ripped*. I was immediately asked to leave.

Movement here was a walk of shame. Movement meant thinking before you speak.

I could speak about so many more stories growing up. Stories and memories that reminded me to not take life too seriously[58]. What all the stories in this chapter (and the ones I have not mentioned) have in common, is the realisation that being able to move, being able to interact and being able to

---

[58] Stories about how at a packed athletics stadium, I walked out of the warmup changerooms, in front of the whole crowd, with a long line of used toilet paper sticking out the back of my running shorts.

freely make a choice are all things we often take for granted. I often tell patients that their pain is a blessing in disguise; it makes you feel alive again. Pain can sometimes remind you that you need to reassess your life. Some people do not have the privilege of experiencing overuse injuries or the pain caused by overuse injuries, instead they experience pain from abuse, judgement, neglect, loneliness, or hatred. In other words, if you are seeing me for treatment, to a certain degree you are privileged.

Movement has, and always will be, a privilege.

Point to ponder: Where can your health improve?

Monaco, Amsterdam,
London

Singapore

John's Hopkins
University, USA

South Africa

The Shire,
New Zealand

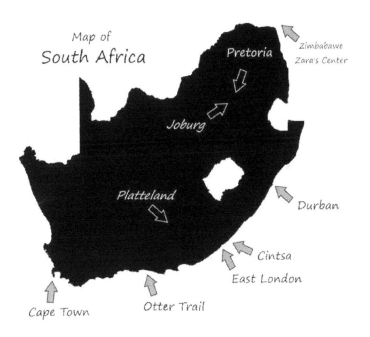

Map of
South Africa

Pretoria

Zimbabawe
Zara's Center

Joburg

Platteland

Durban

Cintsa
East London

Cape Town

Otter Trail

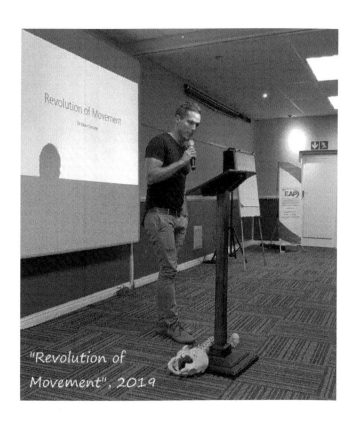

"Revolution of Movement", 2019

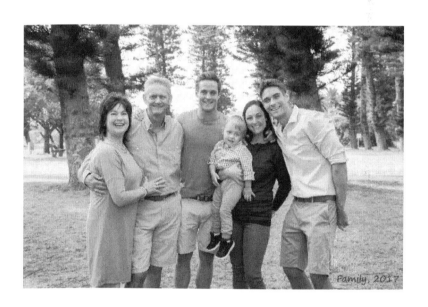

Family, 2017

4 : Moving London

Jon has worked in sales for the last 10 years. Sitting average >8 hours per day. Travels >3000km per month. Sitting is the new smoking - explains his probable disc injury and lack of flexibility.

I graduated from University, said goodbye to Lochner[59] and was appointed to an internship at the sports centre at the University of Pretoria, a popular training centre for aspiring Olympian athletes. I found myself in the presence of some of the biggest names in local sport and some of the top medical minds.

I was a twenty-three year old chiropractic student, insignificant in comparison to the highly qualified lecturers

---

[59] Dr Lochner Slabbert. Incomparable chiropractor, world class rugby player, family man, ultimate man and the most genuine person that I know. He was my big brother throughout my university years. His example is a constant reminder to me to be humbler, serve better and to never take opportunities for granted.

and specialists these courses usually attract. Unaware anyone even knew my name; I was asked to prepare a lecture on "Movement" for the medical doctors specialising in sports medicine. Bear in mind that I was still waiting for my master's dissertation to be marked, so technically I was still a student. What would I have to say that they did not already know? This was surely an error, until it turned out it was not. The lecture was attended by people who were experts in their field, people I held in highest esteem, and yet they came to hear what I had to say. That was a turning point for me, the realisation that I had something to say, that I could educate patients to a healthier life. The ant climbed that molehill quite a few times that day (remember the stutter talking technique?). The ant was rather fit now, but this was still one of the most humbling experiences of my life.

Movement was getting out of my comfort zone. Movement started developing confidence.

MoveMed

If you love what you do, you will never work another day in your life[60]. This stage of learning is called: Adulting.

It was this idea that gave birth to the brand *MoveMed*, which I started in 2013. I believe that both movement and medicine are privileges, wherever you are in the world, but especially in South Africa or any place where shoes, space, safety or health care are hard to come by. One of the only excuses I accept from a patient who does not do exercise is that they do not own shoes, but even then, Zola Budd never

---

[60] I love the cheesiness of this saying. The truth is that we are all human. I do love what I do, but I also have horrible days, days where I have no patience for my patients and days where I do not do any exercise. *But that is O.K.* Do not beat yourself up, start fresh the next day. It would be pointless to stress about a few bad days or weeks, some things you cannot change. Like the past.

ran with shoes on her feet[61].

Here is a shocking statistic for you. According to my brother and the orthopaedic department in which he works in a rural part of South Africa, the hospital has a patient catchment area the size of New Zealand, roughly four million people. All of these people come to one government hospital for certain orthopaedic procedures which are not offered at local clinics. It became so clear to me that movement and medicine are both privileges.

Let us return to my Rule of Sixes.

Beacon Bay Chiropractic

After six years in Durban, I took a locum in my hometown of East London, with Gregg[62], and decided to stay for a while. This ended up being another six-year stint.

In that time, the brilliant Dr Jason Dicks joined us, and we became the Three Musketeers of Beacon Bay. Jason does not know this, but I called him *Strap-on*. It literally looks like his muscles have been strapped onto his body. Eventually his better half, the compassionate Dr Candice Armstrong, joined us and we became the most prominent chiropractic practice in the area.

The practice in East London was called Beacon Bay

---

[61] Yoga, Pilates and Aerobics are other activities which do not require shoes. I should perhaps revise the list of acceptable excuses from patients. Like being a parent. That is legit. Or a patient saying, 'life is busy'. I have learnt that is also legit. Excuses are relative to the individual, and it is not my place to judge someone's reasons, it is however my job to motivate the first small conscious step towards healing.

[62] Dr Gregg Audie. My first boss. Champion spearfisherman and water polo player. We became great work partners and friends. He taught me most of what I know about pain management, how to interact with patients, internal coccyx adjustments and the true meaning of 'no pain, no gain'.

Chiropractic[63]. The building was two kilometres from the beach, and a two hundred-meter commute to my house. I was living the dream, in my view anyway. East London was also where *MoveMed* became a reality. It was here that I registered the trademark for the name and also where I started three satellite MoveMed practices (in three nearby towns in the Eastern Cape).

MoveMed is based on the principle that simply restoring normal movement is the healing mechanism for most of the physical complaints we treat. Our practice was pain-based, and our focus was on myofascial release and adjusting. *Myo* means muscle and *fascia* is the covering of all muscles. An adjustment is a high speed thrust to mobilise a joint that is restricted or not moving. We worked hard, and gave of ourselves physically and mentally, as I believe a doctor and public servant should.

Movement here was livelihood; movement meant learning skills.

East London (Round Two)

In my first year back in East London I did wonder why God had placed me there, but it became obvious as the years passed. One year later my brother was posted to the local government hospital, and so he, my sister-in-law Nicole, and my nephew

---

[63] Dr Ashton Vice. Founder of the practice where Gregg, and eventually I, worked. Now my UK mentor. One of the first chiropractors to practice as a 'true mixer' in South Africa. He taught me to always be true to my patients (in his words 'do not bullsh*t them'). He taught me to always be true to myself (give an honest, undisputable, and researchable health service).

Cameron[64] moved home. Our parents were still living there, and so the whole family was back together. A roller coaster few years followed as little Cammy became ill with what turned out to be a rare genetic disease. I moved into my brother's flatlet to support them (mostly emotionally) for a year. There is a whole chapter on Cammy later that explains it all. It was during this time too that I made some of my closest friends and continued my overseas explorations.

Movement was again gratitude; movement meant overcoming obstacles.

New Zealand (Round Two)

My first taste of UK life was touring internationally with a national indoor cricket team. I was one of their team doctors. My role was to warm up the players and treat bicep strains that were incurred mostly from lifting beer mugs. I suppose this was a true reflection of winter in London.

I arrived from South Africa late in the evening and before I met the team I went to bed. I remember rising early on my first morning there and going for a run at around 5 a.m. There was no one about until I ran past a group of heavily intoxicated individuals walking home after a night out. At the team meeting later on that morning I was met with these same familiar faces, and they instantly gave me hard looks, or so I thought, although it could be possible that they were simply not feeling as fresh as daisies. I was however an honourable teammate and did not mention it, until now, that is. Most importantly, we worked hard and managed to win a world cup medal.

---

[64] Cameron Coetzee. Older brother to Scott. If you ever read this one-day Cam: you are my hero. Without knowing it, his diagnosis will mean his brother will have a better life. A true testimony of something particularly important in life: put others first and try always to give, love and serve more.

Movement was success; movement meant celebration.

Netherlands

The dreams and worldwide explorations continued in 2016. I said goodbye to Weyers[65] and this time was off to the Netherlands. I had already completed part of the International Sports Chiropractic Diploma in the USA, and the nerd inside of me was searching for the next learning challenge. In medicine, you can specialise in numerous different fields. In chiropractic, we do not have too many options. Besides your personal interests where you can do smaller courses, the only other *speciality* in chiropractic would be sports chiropractic or animal chiropractic. My next option was animals. And the only option offered in the chiropractic world would be for dogs and horses. It just so happened that the Netherlands offered a course in canine and equine dry needling. I enquired and a few months later I was on my way.

"Why the long face?" I made that joke every day during my equine dry needling course.

For those of you who do not know how dry needling works, you insert a sterile acupuncture needle into a taut band in the muscle and you manoeuvre around until you elicit a jump response. The muscle will literally jump or twitch, and this is what releases the trigger point. It may sound pretty scientific, but basically the twitch response in the muscle is detected by the nerves, and in the same way as you have a knee jerk reflex, the spinal cord initiates a reflex twitch that relaxes the muscle. A horse's muscles are identical to ours in the way that they react to movement. The muscles need to be warmed up,

---

[65] Weyers Marais. Brilliant designer, family man, life enthusiast and one of my good friends. Weyers and I would have regular hangouts whilst we both lived in East London. We called these 'Dream Sessions'. He calls a spade a spade, as the saying goes, and that's what I need to hear sometimes.

stretched down, hydrated and they suffer fatigue from overuse.

Now when you needle a human, they can swear at you or ask you to kindly stop. A horse, on the other hand, knows only how to buck or kick. During my second month back from doing the course, I had a full day of horses to treat in Queenstown, South Africa. It was nearly the end of the day and the next patient with a long face was Arrow. "*I assure you she is calm*", are the words uttered by every horse owner. As I was taught, I stood next to Arrow's shoulder and leant towards her tight gluteal region (her buttocks). The first few needles were perfect; she gave the ear rotation nod of approval and even did the pushing air through her mouth response. Next thing, I felt a huge jump under my hand and in a flash, I was on my back. Arrow was now half kicking the stable down. I realised that if I had been a few centimetres closer to her hind quarters I could have been in direct contact with the kick, and that would have broken something for sure. The owner was apologetic, but I realised then that I needed to protect the money-maker, which in my case is an able body. I now treat horses only on request.

Needless to say, my passion for treating human beings far outweighs any calling I may hear from the equine world. I did love getting on the open road and experiencing farm life again though. It brought back memories of my grandparents' farm.

Movement can be done in nature; movement meant big muscle jumps.

London

One of my bucket list items was always to watch Usain Bolt live. In 2016 he announced that he was retiring after the 2017 World Championships, I immediately considered selling a kidney to be there. Luckily, that never happened, but I did spend a small fortune on the ticket. And every second - make that every one of the nine seconds - was worth it. To witness that exceptional level of fitness first-hand was unparalleled. To see what an able and fully functional body can do over one hundred meters blew my mind. When the body is fully functional and moving the way it was designed to, it will do everything more efficiently and quicker. Quicker healing. Quicker recovery.

It is no secret that one of the reasons I left South Africa was to try and earn a passport which makes travel easier. Something I would like to give to my children one day. A more important reason was that I wanted to learn a different style of practice, a more efficient way to manage people, and the opportunity to be able to help more people. Even more important than that, I wanted to launch a global education project on Movement, alongside a health coaching program. I also wanted to write this book.

I do not know where MoveMed is going long-term, or who is going to join it, and help expand it. What I do know is that it is not just a chiropractic brand - the avenues of reach are far beyond my clinic room. I am also not certain for how many years I will be calling London home; all I know is that my next move will be a big one. One where I will know what kind of health entity I would like to run one day. As Howard Hughes would say, *"Don't tell me I can't do it, don't tell me it can't be done!"*. You *gotta* dream big[66].

---

[66] A dream, with an achievable plan, becomes reality. I always imagine this. One day you look up the word *move* in the dictionary. In the entry you will see a picture of me. And if you look closer, in the picture I am holding up a copy of this book.

In London, I have noticed a whole new movement dilemma. There is a public transport system second to none, which means people stand and sit a lot. There is also a higher stress profile in the central London business sector. And yet, the average lifespan in the United Kingdom is longer than that in South Africa[67]. Imagine if we could increase healthy years of life in a population who already live longer. The way forward, as I see it, is movement.

Here is one of my many London travel stories. The London Underground, (also known as the Tube), is the train system serving London. I was heading to the lake district in July for a training weekend. The lake district is one the closest things England has to South Africa, a massive beautiful lake, (the name gives it away), surrounded by an ebb and flow of mountain roads and trails. It is ideal cycling and running territory. The only problem was getting my bicycle from New Malden, in South West London, to Rickmansworth, North London, using only public transport. This meant I would need to head straight through Central London. Google maps reckoned the fastest route was on the Underground. So, at 8pm after work, with a backpack and a helmet I started my journey. Still relatively new to the tube, I honestly never knew unfolded bicycles were not allowed on the underground. However, there was a glitch in the system, and I made it through Vauxhall, the first underground entrance I encountered, unnoticed. I now headed on the Victoria line towards Seven Sisters. The second tube I needed to hop onto was the Jubilee line to Stanmore, I needed to change lines at Green Park. I made it through the crowd with a few looks and sneaked onto the tube at Green Park. The intercom went off and I faintly heard the following message over my earphones: *"Would the person who just boarded with a bicycle please get off the train immediately"*. I was not sure if I had heard correctly, so I paused my music and

---

[67] For a number of complex reasons from access to health care to poverty and malnourishment.

waited. Now everyone was looking at me. Then, I heard it again: *"Would the person who just got on with a bicycle please get off the train immediately."*

I realised I was the offending party by the general and subtle smirks of disapproval from my fellow passengers. I poked my head out of the carriage door only to see the train driver at the front of the train with his finger curling, indicating I should go on over. I was quite frankly exhausted by now and only needed to make it on to the last train for the evening. I needed a lucky break. As I approached the man, all I could say was: *"Please Sir, I need your help."* He was quite shocked; I could see him ease back in his posture (I am sure he was used to drunk or simply rude people causing havoc on his line.) I explained that I was new to London from South Africa, and that I never knew bicycles were not allowed. I explained that I was one change away from my destination, and that it would be counter-productive to go back now. He immediately said I could put my bike and myself in the driver's cab (the historically correct name for the cockpit of a train in the London Underground) and ride with him in the front to my next stop, which was Finchley Road. What a relief.

He took the opportunity to show me what the underground looks like from his viewpoint by switching every single light in the driver's cab off and allowing us to follow the 150 (or so) year-old wormhole. He was clearly old school; he told me that he had done time in the military before becoming a train driver when the system was still manual driving. Now of course, it is all automated. He told me that no normal civilian would have seen what he had just shown me. We briefly chatted and then we sat there for eleven minutes and five stops enjoying this rare treat.

Movement can open doors.

Even now, the public transport system in London; the buses, the tube and the trains, and the management thereof boggles my mind. Something I have started doing is stretching and squatting on trains. You will see later that too much sitting is not great for your back. I have therefore started sitting into a deep squat on trains for the duration of my journey. The looks I have received to date have expressed the general sentiment that I am peculiar. On one occasion, a group of young lads looked at me, and one mumbled something to himself. I agreed with him in my head as I considered that my squat form was *not bad* and gave him an appreciative nod. Little did I know that what he was actually said was: *knobhead*. I of course realised this after the fact.

Movement is humiliating at times.

Your Majesty

Having grown up in a society where inequality is stark, and poverty is normal for most. I am grateful for the privilege and opportunities I have had and try actively not to take things for granted. It is extremely easy to be humble in South Africa. When people have asked me what my life was like in South Africa, I have said that it is my ideal home. The weather is perfect. My family are there. The lifestyle is second to none.

Take East London as an example. My average day was as follows: Treat patients 6 a.m. to 3 p.m. (yes, we started that early, this was something else that Gregg taught me). And the afternoons and evenings were for anything and everything else - surfing (weather permitting), exercising, visiting my family, friends, or even a sneaky road trip to Cintsa. This lifestyle was bolstered by copious amounts of sunshine. I have since realised that I will one day need to live in a place as sunny as 'home'.

My favourite place for a holiday is a small stretch of coastline called Cintsa. It offers surfable waves, reefs and beach breaks, heavy barrels at graveyards, tidal pools for children, fishing and spearfishing alike, long white sandy beaches, trail running and hiking. The weather is wonderful all year round. This paradise is nevertheless a sharp contrast to the everyday life of your average South African.

It is against this backdrop that I must share a glass shattering moment that took place whilst I was making my way to a course I was attending in Windsor. It would take me an hour and forty-five-minutes on buses and trains to get there. One major difference between South Africa and first world countries, is that public transport is used primarily by low income earners. I was privileged to drive a car in South Africa and had no idea what it meant to have to rely on public transport. Sometimes, rarely, my domestic helper Kutela would arrive late for work. This could put me out by ten minutes. At the time, the notion of anyone being late for anything was simply unacceptable in my mind and I would feel annoyed by the delay. I mean, leave earlier Kutela. Right?

On the day I was attending my course in Windsor, I calculated that I would need to leave two hours before the course to make it on time, provided that the trains and buses played their part. And why would they not? I arrived at Windsor Station with my friend Mitch who was also attending the course, and the buses were not in-service because of road works near the Queen's house. I mean, how inconvenient Your Majesty. The traffic was gridlocked and therefore Uber would take even longer, and Bolt had no drivers that far out of London. Our last option was to walk the four kilometres from the train station to the course venue. Mitch is a power lifter, and he often says I am crazy to go on even a five kilometre run, so this was a tall order for Mitch. He was not impressed when I said, "Bru, we need to walk, and fast. Because if we are late, we are wasting their time!".

We arrived ten minutes late and it was a great walk, for me anyway. Mitch is a strong lad and he has big muscles. He complained that he had chaffed his inner thighs. I asked him to please not say that out loud ever again.

It was somewhere along the walk I realised that we were going to be late and there was absolutely nothing I could do to prevent that. In that instant, a cloud of shame filled my head.

How many times had I reprimanded Kutela and told her to leave earlier when she said there was a problem with an already inefficient and dangerous taxi service in SA? The only difference between her and me is the fact that I managed to be late in a city renowned for its efficient and reliable transport system.

My first visit home after moving to the UK was in February 2020. I apologised to Kutela for my ignorance and she was gracious. We laughed together about it over a cup of instant coffee.

Movement that day meant eating humble pie, in large slices.

And there you have it, a few fitful pages out of my memory bank to share some lessons learnt, and how 'movement' feeds my perspective on life and 'being' in this world. Let us move (on). That is hopefully one of the reasons you have this book in your hands, after all.

Point to ponder: Be kind, you never know what someone else is going through.

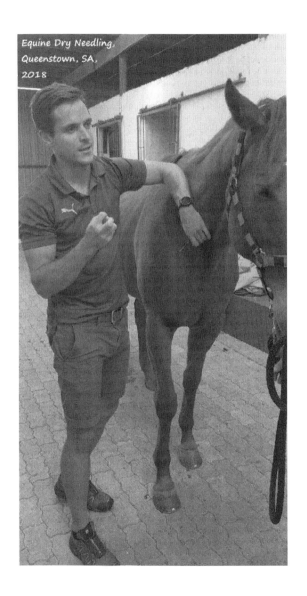

Equine Dry Needling, Queenstown, SA, 2018

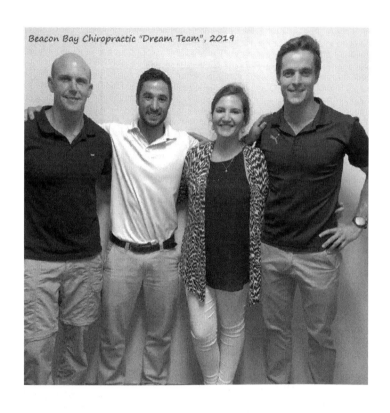

Beacon Bay Chiropractic "Dream Team", 2019

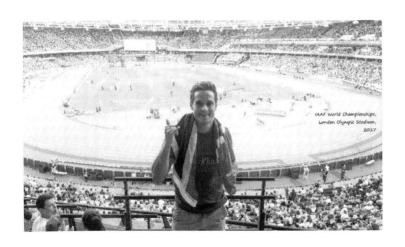

IAAF World Championships,
London Olympic Stadium,
2017

5 : Moving Concepts

Jon runs six days a week with one rest day.
Core and flexibility "average". He has not
heard the word "Proprioception" before. Sleeps
on average 6 hours per night. Diet is high in
sugar and refined carbs. Alcohol not an issue.
So much room for improvement. This is
positive.

There is no "I" in *health*, but there is "heal". That saying has become meaningful for me as it summarizes how I view health (and being unhealthy). Health can be understood as a simple seesaw analogy, and one which is tilting in the favour of healing. It is black and white; if you are not healing, or in a healing environment, you are deteriorating.

There is so much information available literally at our fingertips, along with statistics and statements that we accept without really thinking about them. You will see the concepts described in this chapter creeping in throughout the book and how they play a role in our health, exercise and healing.

This stage of learning is called: Educate the patient.

Before you can heal, you need to ask yourself if you are willing to give up the things that made you unhealthy in the first place. That is the first step of healing, a conscious choice[68].

The second step is to identify the stressors which made you unhealthy. In my experience, these stressors can be summarized as excess stress and excess inflammation. You need to identify where excess stress is in your life and where excess inflammation is coming from. This step often includes treatment. If you have lost function in a joint, muscle or nerve, a *Neural Re-Education* protocol[69] may help restore the lost function.

'Excess' stress and 'excess' inflammation is relative. Everyone will respond differently to different amounts of either. We shall see later exactly what classifies as stress and inflammation. However, for now, understanding that we need less of both of them is good enough.

The third step of healing is to adopt a lifestyle which will prevent them from re-occurring. This is also known as a recovery-driven lifestyle, which includes clean eating, Zone 2 exercise and maintaining a positive mindset.

My job as a Health Coach is addictive in the sense that every case offers a unique challenge. As you saw with my New

---

[68] I am of course not referring to those instances in which people are suffering from rare genetic disorders, cancer, immunodeficiencies, and illnesses alike that do not discriminate between healthy or unhealthy bodies.

[69] This word has popped up a few times already. If had to summarize what treatment I deliver for a living, the answer is *Neural Re-Education* protocol. A simple concept of teaching the body to move the best it can. Joints and muscles are controlled by the brain; hence it is called *Neural*. How much movement you can restore is of course relative to how much damage has already been done (and many other factors you will see in this book). But the bottom line is that it is never too late to start.

York marathon, I love a challenge. The work is addictive because every patient is different, with a different set of goals and different stressors, and my desire to help people better themselves is why I went into healthcare in the first place. When you make a breakthrough in someone's life and they offer a heartfelt *thank you,* for simply restoring their ability to perform a mundane task; it is humbling. I think it is this humility, that you can have a small part to play in someone else's joy, that is the real addiction.

My job is to facilitate those steps that help create a healing environment. It may be in phase one to remind you that you are strong enough, that you have it in you. My job also always involves step two, where, together, we find out what stressors are affecting your body - physical, mental, emotional, chemical or spiritual. Finally, my job also involves phase three in motivating you to continue your preventative measures, whichever those are that have been personalized to your condition, and the physical maintenance of your body to keep it moving in the way it was designed to move.

There are a few basic concepts to understand about movement and how they pertain to our health. These are encapsulated in an approach I have termed *MoveMed*, where movement itself is medicine.

CONCEPT ONE: Move how you were designed to move[70].

If there was one purpose for this book, this would be it. All the big themes in this book span from this idea: *How do we move the way we were designed to move?*

If you look at the spine and pelvis, there is absolutely no way they are designed to be stationary. The pelvic bones are two huge weight bearing bones (as seen in the picture at the end of this chapter), and with the sacrum, they make up the pelvis. From your head to your sacrum, there are 24 vertebrae (in most people): seven neck vertebrae, twelve midback vertebrae (to which the ribs also attach) and five lower back vertebrae. Any engineer would suggest that the size of a joint dictates how much movement that joint should take, (which makes sense if you think about it logically). Sacroiliac joints are the two moveable joints between the pelvic bones and the sacrum. Relatively speaking, they are huge. The 24 vertebrae above the sacrum are tiny in comparison. The size and orientation of the facet joints, (the joints between the vertebrae), suggest that they are meant to swivel and transfer weight, and not to lift it. With this concept we introduce the fact that we start to lift with our spines, (as opposed to lifting with our hips and pelvis) and translate the weight evenly through all the vertebrae.

This is the most important movement concept, as it affects all the others. *Flexibility* is needed to maintain movement in your pelvis. *Core strength* is needed to support the spine when

---

[70] I am aware that some people may fundamentally disagree with this question of 'design'. I am a creationist, but this principle is wholly applicable if you are an evolutionist. Imagine the first human who would have evolved from an ape. Ape and human alike, if you could not move to hunt or feed yourself, natural selection took over and you died. So, when I speak about moving how you were *designed* to move, it should be clear that the mechanics of our pelvis and spine are engineeringly designed for a certain type of movement as you will see. And irregularities with this movement causes dysfunction of many kinds.

it is taking load against gravity. *Proprioception* is needed to control the joints subconsciously. *Chiropractic intervention* is often needed to restore movement mechanically in joints that stop moving. *Normal movement* is needed to decrease inflammation in joints.

CONCEPT TWO : Create a healing environment.

Being healthy means having an internal healing environment. An internal healing environment means that stress and inflammation are low enough to promote the body to heal. Think of the analogy of a seesaw again. Stress and inflammation are the opposite of healing. Too much of those, and the body cannot attain an internal healing environment[71].

There are things we can do that tilt that seesaw in our favour. Exercise, NRE, clean eating and recovery - to name a few.

---

[71] In the right environment, we either grow or die. I witnessed this at university. It was 2nd year biochemistry, and the class were all given our own Petri dishes. This is a shallow transparent lidded dish, containing a hard gel (a nutritious medium providing the perfect growing environment) that biologists use to culture cells, such as bacteria or fungi. We were instructed to swab any surface, like the desk or chair, and to make a pattern on the gel surface with the contaminated swab, and in a few weeks, we would see how the bacteria had grown exactly where the swab had touched. The guys in the class, albeit immature, agreed to draw the shape of male genitals in our dishes. A few weeks later, one dish in particular had grown so much that it displaced its lid. It turns out, instead of drawing a penis, a certain someone had swabbed his.

CONCEPT THREE : Not moving could cause disease[72].

Over the last seven years I have realised that the lack of movement, inactivity, is a large risk factor for most of the mechanical injuries that I treat. Lack of exercise is the largest risk factor for chronic diseases. They are the mutual denominators. Movement does not only pertain to physical activity; movement also relates physiologically and psychologically to the body.

A joint does not need to be injured to stop moving. The physical act of not moving will signal to the brain that you do not need to use that joint anymore, and the system will stop using it. Once that has become the new norm, we need to teach the system what normal movement is. One way to do that is with a *Neural Re-Education* protocol.

The body craves movement. There is a positive spinoff to movement that is both conscious and subconscious. I believe it is in our genes, like the beating of our hearts, the rhythm of movement is music to the soul. I have read a few articles that have agreed that it takes 21 days to form a new habit. I have found it takes no more than 17 days for the new activity to feel completely normal. That is a little over two weeks. Half a month. That is all it takes to make a start.

CONCEPT FOUR : You cannot fix mechanics with medicine.

Take this case.

---

[72] As a reference to the movie *DEAD POET'S SOCIETY*, do not become a member of the *Dead Movement Society*.

August 2016

Katniss Everdeen, a 17-year-old female presented to the Clinic. She is a smart and diligent young girl who enjoys playing games outdoors.

Patient presents with severe lower sacral pain after two days prior having fallen and landed with her tailbone on the corner of an outside bench. Patient now cannot sit.

It was obvious we needed to rule out a broken coccyx. X-rays were taken. The lazy diagnosis was Coccydynia (the medical term for pain in your coccyx), more specifically the Lateral Pelvic X-ray showed an internally dislocated coccyx with no fracture (the coccyx is now bent inwards).

Katniss's treatment options were to wait for six weeks in pain (eventually the coccyx would fuse in its dislocated position) or to have an internal procedure to relocate the tailbone involving gloves, medical K-Y Jelly (a water based lubricant) and a terribly invasive internal procedure.

The next day Katniss arrived at the Clinic with both her parents. They watched as I performed the delicate procedure on their daughter who was curled up in a foetal position. Eye contact with her parents was avoided while I performed the internal procedure to manipulate the tail bone back into place. Sweat was dripping from my forehead[73].

The good-to-knows:

ONE. The procedure was a success and Katniss could sit, pain-free, three days later. Sometimes, movement is the only medicine.

TWO. When it is a mechanical problem, no pill will get a

---

[73] The grip used to grab the coccyx is that of a 'six-pack grip'. In South Africa, beers or cans of soft drinks can be purchased in packs of six, which are all tightly concealed in plastic wrapping. If your hands are full of other groceries, the only way to pick up the six-pack would be to push your finger through the plastic wrapping between the beers and bend it inside as to get a grip. That is the coccyx contact needed for the adjustment. Let it never be said that I would not go the extra mile for a patient.

restricted joint moving again.

This is the dilemma: you have severe muscle spasm that is protecting a joint strain or a disc. The body is protecting the joint. A spasm like that will often not respond to drugs such as muscle relaxants. The essential thing for that muscle spasm would be to get the joint that the involved muscle moves, moving. Yes, the joint is most likely inflamed, but it is exacerbated by the spasm. We show the body that the joint can still move, and that spasm falls asleep.

Medical doctors are undeniably essential for society, so, this is in no way a criticism of doctors, but the fact is that medicine will not change gross mechanics. It will help for pain, no doubt. But pain is often the last symptom to come and normally the first to leave. That is why it is so essential to treat function and not only pain.

Other rhetorical questions you can ask yourself here. *If my chronic prescription drugs alone worked, would I need to fill a prescription? Or, if my body was not lacking paracetamol, why did I take it?*

We need to restore normal movement, physically, and re-educate the body about what normal movement feels like.

CONCEPT FIVE : If you do not use it, you lose it.

Our brain has one major function – to navigate adaptable and complex movements. Take the koala as an example. It has one of the smallest brains (in proportion to skull cavity) in the animal kingdom. Why? Over time, koalas have changed their lifestyle to live only in and around eucalyptus trees. They do not need to move much now. It is clear - the less you physically move, the less you need your brain. Consequently, it will shrink.

Yes. If you do not use it (brain), you will lose it (shrink).

The best way that I know to use your brain is exercise. Every time a joint or muscle moves, a specific part of the brain is stimulated.

Similarly, I had X-rays of my teeth during a routine dental check-up. I found out that I do not have wisdom teeth. Not even undescended ones. When I asked the dentist why, he said that he is seeing this phenomenon more often these days. The reason is that most of the food we eat these days is softer, more often processed, and cooked. This means that we as humans have no need for late developmental wisdom teeth to help grind hard unprocessed and raw foods. You see if we do not use it, genetically and down a generation, we lose it.

CONCEPT SIX : Muscles do *not* have their own memory

Unlike an octopus, we do not have brains in our limbs, therefore, it is impossible to *remember* anything in our arms or legs. But it is true that once you learn how to do something physical - whether a squat or a leg balance exercise - it becomes easier and easier to perform it without thinking about the movement it involves. It really does *feel* as if your body remembers how to do the movement. There is a point when the body seems to effortlessly perform the movement without conscious activity. The reality is that the activity is happening in our brains.

This concept, however, is not so singular. The previous chapters explored all the different things movement can mean. These were less biological and more experiential. In other words, movement can be whatever you experience it to be. In phenomenology, it is called 'embodiment' or 'embodied knowledge'. Your body remembers even when it feels like your mind may not.

Sometimes our bodies respond to a sound, a smell, a touch in a way our minds do not seem to have control over - a visceral experience (getting goose bumps when someone speaks of something stirring, repulsive or beautiful). Or *butterflies* in your stomach thinking about someone you love. I know this is a medical book, but when you look at the body less as a culmination of cells, organs, parts and more as a vessel that interacts, engages and experiences the world - the body does remember things the mind 'forgets' or chooses to block out (one example is people with PTSD).

In my scope of practice, clinically how I treat patients and for this book's purpose, I care mostly about restoring normal movement. The other clinical benefits stem from that. *Neural Re-Education* or NRE; we attempt to *neurally* re-educate normal movement. But more on this later.

CONCEPT SEVEN : Muscles and joints need to be re-educated

Are you *going* through life or are you *growing* through it? You need to be learning, adapting, reacting and repeating.

Any joint or muscle needs to be re-educated concerning what normal movement is after any injury. It is something I must explain every time I see a patient.

Any old injury, even an injury incurred during childhood, would have left the body with an abnormal muscle memory. Here is one example. A patient, a 40-year-old, man fell and fractured his pelvis when he was eleven years old. At that time, (roughly 30 years ago), protocol for a fractured pelvis was six weeks of bed rest. That was it. When that patient stood up for the first time in six weeks, the body would naturally have shifted weight onto the opposite leg, as a compensatory mechanism, and that would have never been corrected. Now, aged 40, he has severe hip joint degenerative changes as a result of the compensation pattern that was never rehabilitated to normal motion and movement.

You have seen this word many times already, but it is called

Neural Re-Education[74] and there is a lot more about this later. How long will this re-education take? Around six weeks. If Michael Jordan strained his hamstring, it would take around six weeks at the least to regenerate, heal and develop. If you are 80 years old, it would take much longer - up to five years. The point is that long term healing will not happen overnight. It needs habitual movement, coupled with good recovery, to heal and re-educate normal movement.

CONCEPT EIGHT : Things get worse before they get better.

I always explain to patients that, "Tomorrow, it may feel like I have punched you". This has happened so often. On numerous occasions, a patient has come to me to treat neck pain, and while I am tending to the neck, the lower back flares up.

There are a few reasons for this:

Firstly, the body always focuses on *its worst* area. As pain decreases in this area, the brain can focus on other areas where perhaps there was no pain before, because the body was focussing on the worst area.

Secondly, take the neck as an example. During treatment, advice would normally be given on correct postures. If the patient starts to sit and stand differently, the lower back is loaded in a different way, and therefore joints and muscles take a load which they are not used to taking. These structures fatigue and become symptomatic, appearing as if we have caused a new pain, when all we have done is decrease the primary pain.

---

[74] This word is appearing again. NRE. *Neural Re-Education*. Start getting used to it. These two words summarize one of the most important treatment tools I can offer to my patients; physically being able to work with patients and teaching their bodies how to move properly again.

I always warn patients that this might happen. I remember clearly having forgotten to remind a patient that they may be sore after treatment. And she was the one in many that had an unbelievably painful reaction to the treatment. No matter how I tried to explain over the phone that pain after treatment was normal, nothing helped. *Lesson learnt* .

Third, the body is brilliant in the manner in which it compensates. It is like an onion. As you remove one layer, there is a whole new set of compensations. For example, if I had to adjust or mobilise a joint that has been locked or restricted for years, the pain will increase for a few days as the body experiences a new range of motion or a new joint load. Simultaneously, the opposite side of the body starts to pain as the body was always compensating there but the symptoms were always felt on the injured side.

Often, *pain is gain*[75], and *to avoid pain, you need to maintain (movement)*.

CONCEPT NINE : Stop 'cracking' your own neck.

The first question most people ask me is, "Is it bad to crack my own neck?"

Let us all agree that it feels good when you crack your own neck, but please stop. What is happening when one does this, is that unstable joints are being made more unstable. The body is expressing its need for more movement and cracking one's own neck only gives a temporary relief. It only moves the joints that are easy to move. The joints that are restricted or *stuck* remain that way.

That is where a chiropractor comes in, to move joints that

---

[75] And also, while we are rhyming, west is best. This is something you learn quickly growing up in South Africa. On the east coast, in surfing terms, the east wind makes choppy unsurfable waves. East is least. West wind brings the clean breaking waves.

the patients cannot move themselves[76]. It is also common for a patient who has participated in a *Neural Re-Education* protocol, to have less of an urge to click their own neck.

All that tells me is that we have restored movement in the joints that originally were not moving. The body does not produce the *feeling* that it needs to increase movement for itself. Therefore, the answer to the question is *yes* and do not do it[77].

CONCEPT TEN : Pills only mask symptoms

I am not in principle opposed to taking medication for joint and muscular pain. I have plenty to say about medication that is over-prescribed when it is simply not warranted. There is a reason that the opioid crisis climaxed when it did. There is a reason that a certain pharmaceutical giant had to pay back over $500 million in the first trial for the destruction wrought by prescription painkillers. (True story, ask Google.)

Here is something to ponder on. The body ingests a foreign particle like a bacteria or virus. In response, the brain raises the body's core temperature (called a fever), to create a healing

---

[76] Everyone always asks if I am going to break their neck when I adjust it. Thank you, Jackie Chan. The truth is that, unlike martial arts movies, chiropractors contact the neck with our fingers. I would never intentionally break my own finger. Secondly, and this may sound controversial; If I broke someone's neck with my finger, that would be extremely helpful, as it would indicate a pathological fracture and the patient most likely would have had a cancer that we never knew about. Thirdly, when it comes to elderly patients, the adjustment should change to a gentle mobilization.

[77] Whenever I adjust someone's neck, I always explain that they may hear gunshots. To explain that, the inner hollow chamber of your ear sits inside the skull bone that lies directly on top of your first neck vertebrae. You can hear your fingers click a distance away from your head. If you have never had your neck adjusted, just imagine the gunshots you will hear if that click happened inside your ear. It is a very satisfying bang. *That's what she said.*

environment for the body. The body is then given a pill to ingest to lower this fever. The brain must be wondering *what is going on here.* Similarly, the body is physically injured. The brain initiates an inflammatory response to create a healing environment. Again, the body ingests a pill to lower this inflammation. Once more the brain is left bewildered.

This happens again and again, and eventually the body will adapt to this counter response. Ultimately our natural defence mechanism weakens, becomes less potent or shuts down. This explains why people become sick so often - the fever response is less efficient as it is always being dampened by pills. This same principle applies to our core muscle activations, proprioception and many other important body functions. *If we don't use them, we lose them.*

In both scenarios, movement would be beneficial. Especially in the latter case. A painfully swollen joint or muscle will benefit from light movement, even in the initial acute phase. It makes sense to allow all the new connective tissue, including scar tissue, to form in lines that are congruent with the movement of that joint or muscle. If we do not do that, scar tissue will form in a ball, and this is merely a nidus for future injury as the adjacent tissue is put under stress.

CONCEPT ELEVEN : If you do not move, eventually you will pay someone to move you.

This, basically, summarizes my job. Patients have to some degree lost the ability to move a joint, or a muscle, or a ligament and my job is to restore normal movement.

CONCEPT TWELVE : Move like the four-year-old you.

Let us take a different look at moving the way you were designed to move. An example is the way a four-year-old performs a squat - a perfect deep squat, maintaining the three curves of the spine, whilst bearing weight through the heels. It utilises perfect activation of the posterior muscle chain. The rarity of being able to achieve this as we get older is an example of how we lose our primal posture and integrated movement patterns purely through 21st century lifestyles such as sitting, driving and stationary standing.

Here is a fun fact. There is almost no low back pain in childhood. I have not managed to find a single study of this. Why is that though? It is because of less exposure to life's stressors. Children have not sat or stressed for long enough yet. They are still moving the way the body was designed to move, stressing the body in the way it was designed to be stressed and recovering in the manner the body knows how to recover. It seems children are creating and maintaining an internal healing environment.

CONCEPT THIRTEEN : Underuse is worse than overuse.

I would rather treat a patient with an overuse injury than a patient with an underuse injury any day. An overuse injury tells me that the patient is at least moving, which means there will be a good vascular supply to the problem area. The more blood that reaches the injured area, the faster the healing will be, as it is blood that brings oxygen and substances needed to repair injuries.

Injuries that occur as a lack of movement, such as prolonged disc pressures or joint strains, are often chronic and even the pain aspect of those injuries lasts longer than that of overuse injuries. Neural Re-Education also takes longer[78].

CONCEPT FOURTEEN : Change is inevitable, choose to be on the right side of it.

The human body is astonishing. Some days at work I sit back and think what a privilege it is to be able to see first-hand how the body works. With all the available technologies, is it not incredible that scientists are still making new discoveries about the body, and the brain in particular?

If you push the body's limits, the body will have to induce an adaption that will allow it to perform that task more efficiently in the future. This adaption, with quality and adequate recovery, is called healing. This is the principle that is applied to fitness and health (more on this later).

In other words, when your body becomes ill, it develops protective mechanisms like antibodies to fight said illness in the future. Similarly, athletes push their bodies, their bodies adapt, and the athlete moves faster. Both scenarios are dependent on the quality of recovery.

CONCEPT FIFTEEN : Movement can sometimes be stationary.

This is not a statement designed to rival Newton's theories. Earlier I gave the example of squatting on a train. To refresh your memory, instead of sitting or standing on a bus or train, I try a classic Asian continent deep squat. This movement

---

[78] *I'm just coming in for a realignment.* Or. *Please put my hip back in again.* How many times have I heard those words before? I understand it makes logical sense that you get 'realigned', and you move better. But it is not true. A joint is not simply consistently out of place or dislocated, the joint is simply not moving. If it was dislocated, you would most likely be in hospital.

standard is stationary to an observer, but a series of primal muscle activations happen to hold your body in that position.

No matter how silly it looks, and if you can, start squatting wherever possible.

CONCEPT SIXTEEN : Knees only bend.

Your knee joint is a simple hinge joint. It is designed to bend and extend. Where you are right now you can bend your knee and straighten it again and you will see it only has that one movement.

Quickly cast your attention to your ankle. It moves in all directions, try it, you can make circles with your ankle. You can even write letters of the alphabet on the floor using the movement of your ankle. Now quickly focus your attention on your hip. It also moves in different directions, any directions, called rotational movements.

As you can see, the knee joint is the link between your hip and your ankle. Knee injuries and knee pain are extremely simple to treat when your goal is to restore movement. If you focus on the pain inside the knee, you will only ever have temporary relief. The pain always returns.

You need to treat the mechanics if you want a longstanding solution to your knee pain. Correct the movement. It is vitally important that the knee bends only in a straight line. When the knee begins to twist while you are walking, running, cycling or bending, that is when you experience pain. You feel pain because the knee is not designed to twist or bend to the side. You feel pain because with abnormal movements come abnormal forces through the knee. And with abnormal forces comes inflammation.

Treatment is easy, correct the movement. You need full motion of your hip and pelvis to allow your knee to land in such a way that it needs to bend only in a straight line. You also need full control and stability of your ankle and the arch of your foot. If you do not have this full control, the ankle can collapse. If the ankle collapses, all your weight goes through the inside of the knee as opposed to evenly through it.

Keep it simple. Release the hip and show stretches to increase or maintain pelvis movement (flexibility), restore movement in the pelvis (NRE protocol), regain control of your ankle (proprioception) and your pelvis (core).

CONCEPT SEVENTEEN : Put your own oxygen mask on first.

Always put your own oxygen mask on before helping someone else. This is such a simple yet vital phrase we hear from air hosts and hostesses. But have you ever slowed down to think about why they say that? If you are not alive, you cannot help anyone. The afterlife cannot use your help.

You need to put your own health first. I had to learn this too and have had to keep reminding myself. The giving tree can only give so much.

When I am booked off work, I cannot help anyone in person. There is no way I can help people if I am sick, and sickness is not only physical, it is emotional, mental and psychological. How can I motivate someone to change their lifestyle for the better if I am not in a mentally sound place? I am human and sometimes I put on a performance worthy of an Oscar, but when I do, I know I need to assess where I am lacking oxygen. I may need more sleep. I may need to eat cleaner. My body may require more rest. I might need to apologize to someone and ask their forgiveness. I need to fill my cup before I can pour it out to help others. Our giving potential is greatest when we are both alive and well - not only when we are alive.

When I do get sick it is usually from man flu or that one time, I had hepatitis. Oh, and Covid-19. Men experience worse flu symptoms than women[79].

CONCEPT EIGHTEEN : Keep it simple.

After everything you have just read, if you only remember one thing, let it be this. There is so much information out there. So much information in here. So much new information every day. So many 'experts' that know everything about your life and your health and how to perfect these things.

You can even diagnose yourself on the internet. You can find programs online to fix your spine, your mind or your sexual life. You even can find reasons on Google for or against things like drinking water, drinking alcohol or eating fast food like McDonald's.

So, let us just KISS[80]. My mom always said, 'Just kiss it better'. This has never been truer in my life and in my practice. KISS means 'Keep it simple (and be) smart'. If you are experiencing joint or muscular pain, do not rush to the neurosurgeon, apply heat, or ice and get an appointment with a recommended, or trusted, manual therapist of any kind. If you are unfit, start with the basics of core activations and stretching. If your diet is horrible, start with cutting out one bad item of food at a time. If you have a headache, stretch, apply heat, and go to bed. *Keep it simple.*

Everything in this book is free. Everything is designed to make a lifestyle that is sustainable.

In keeping it simple, here is a summary of the major concepts to understand when it comes to healing, health, and medicine. Keep these in the back of your head whenever you

---

[79] I am actually being serious. Anatomically, most male's skulls are larger than female's skulls, and therefore have more fever receptors. Consequently, the perceived distress of the common cold, or flu, is worse.

[80] Offence is taken, not given. The original meaning of KISS was 'Keep it simple, Stupid'. We changed that to 'Keep it simple (and be) smart'. It is less offensive.

go for a consultation. These are the golden nuggets of health. If you understand these, you could save lots of money and add healthy years to your life.

ONE: Move how you were designed to move.
TWO: Create a healing environment.
THREE: Not moving could cause disease.
FOUR: You cannot fix mechanics with medicine.
FIVE: If you do not use it, you lose it.
SIX: Muscles do *not* have their own memory.
SEVEN: Muscles and joints need to be re-educated.
EIGHT: Things get worse before they get better.
NINE: Stop cracking your own neck.
TEN: Pills only mask symptoms.
ELEVEN: If you do not move, eventually you will pay someone to move you.
TWELVE: Move like the 4-year-old you.
THIRTEEN: Underuse is worse than overuse.
FOURTEEN: Change is inevitable, choose to be on the right side of it.
FIFTEEN: Movement can sometimes be stationary.
SIXTEEN: Knees are only meant to bend.
SEVENTEEN: Put your own oxygen mask on first.
EIGHTEEN: Keep it simple.

Point to ponder: Where are you lacking some *oxygen* in your life?

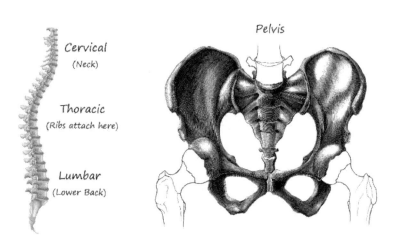

Cervical
(Neck)

Thoracic
(Ribs attach here)

Lumbar
(Lower Back)

Pelvis

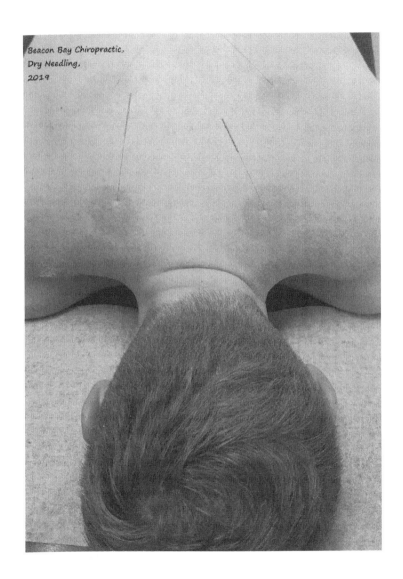

Beacon Bay Chiropractic,
Dry Needling,
2019

117

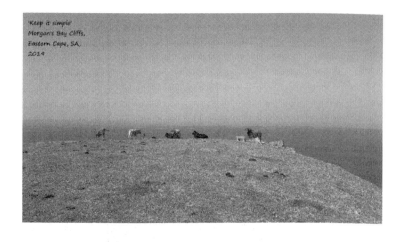

'Keep it simple'
Morgan's Bay Cliffs,
Eastern Cape, SA,
2019

6 : Good Posture and Slipping Discs

Jon was diagnosed with ADHD at the age of 6.
Turns out sugar was the underlying cause, and
he was weaned off Ritalin by the age of 9.
Significant childhood trauma includes a tib-fib
fracture from football aged 13, repaired
surgically with an external fixator and titanium
plates. Plates removed age 14. *Sugar - the
Darth Vader of nutrition.*

H omo erectus. Our own species is literally defined
as being *upright humans*. So why has sitting
become a normal state of being for so many of us,
to the point that we now track our steps on our Fitbits and
Apple watches to account for the time that we are not sitting?
Medical insurance companies also offer incentives for their
members to achieve certain 'steps' (goals), as though investing
in one's health is not enough motivation. We need someone to
dangle a carrot, or perhaps rather, a free double ristretto venti

half-soy non-fat decaf frappuccino from Starbucks, to get us out of our seats! In my opinion, the benefits of having a good posture are reward enough, and here are some reasons why.

Mentally, a good posture has a positive psychological spin off. A good posture emits an outward confident demeanour, and if we *look good, we feel good*, that is for sure.

Physically, a good posture will add healthy years to your spine and body by decreasing the mechanical stress coefficient within your spinal column. In other words, less wear and tear. Good posture is also important for balance. We will see more of this in the chapter *Proprioception*.

Spiritually, a good posture opens us up to a place of meditation and allows for deep breathing. One's posture can also be a window to the soul - it can give expression to the attitudes of our hearts, shame, dejection, regret and pride, but also humility, hope, acceptance, determination.

The clinical benefits I have seen of good posture are less low back pain, fewer headaches, an increase in energy and lung capacity, as well as improved digestion.

Abnormal postures are often an indication of an abnormally functioning nervous system. The body sometimes puts itself in a position to take physical tension off the neurological system. An example of this is how the body, if it is experiencing sciatica down one leg, will move its centre of gravity to the opposite side (observed as a pelvic rotation). Or how in disc patients, the body will not allow itself to bend forward or bare down (such as a cough or a sneeze). Remember that nerves do not stretch, or at least nowhere near as much as muscles, tendons and ligaments do.

You do not need a perfect posture as of right now. Sometimes all you need is a *change* of posture. A different *neural* stimulation. The body's naturally good posture expression will show itself eventually. Of course, sometimes to get there you will need some physical interventions as you have just seen in the *Moving Concepts*[81].

Would you like to see what current modern lifestyles do to our natural postures? Here is something practical. Wherever you are, take a moment and stand up. Now let your arms hang at your sides. What do you notice? If your thumbs point inward towards your body, that is what the 21st century lifestyle does to our posture: the pectoral/ chest muscles shorten, and this internally rotates our arms, and our thumbs point inwards. In a primal and anatomically normal posture, our thumbs would stay pointing outwards.

What if you could make your movement more efficient or even just less painful? As a health care practitioner, I have been captivated by this question for the past thirteen years, because while transportation and technology have brought about a world of sitting and stationary productivity, it has come at the cost of our naturally occurring physical mobility and our bodies' need for movement.

Bobbleheads

The most visually friendly image I can use to describe a good posture to you is that of a bobblehead (those often ridiculous looking collector's dolls with oversized heads that bob around). Your spine should be orientated in such a way that your head balances on your shoulders like a bobblehead. The head should balance itself gently above your shoulders without the use of major muscle support from the neck.

Some animals are designed to have a default forward head carriage, like a horse for instance. And did you know that a horse can sleep standing up, because the biomechanics of its

---

[81] There is a saying in politics. Never let a good crisis go to waste. If your health or posture is in crisis, that just means that you have room for improvement. You have health potential, and I believe it was Winston Churchill who said that continuous effort is the key to unlocking our potential. Baby steps.

neck hold its head in position? Humans were not designed that way, therefore every second that our head is not above our shoulders, certain muscles activate to keep it from dropping further.

A fine movement, like one where your head moves forward, would activate deep neck muscles that are premeditated to hold your head in that position. It is quite simple; if your head leans forward, as it does in the action of looking at a screen or cell phone for hours, there is no way that the relatively small deep neck muscles can hold up your head. Your body will therefore recruit bigger muscles that are able to produce the power needed for that activity. Just like the way I recruited muscles in the latter part of my New York Marathon.

Remember, power muscles are not designed for postural work such as long stationary postures, and eventually they will fatigue. It is here that we meet an old friend called, *Stiff Neck*.

A good posture becomes attainable only when the mechanics of the body are under perfect control. Remember, *we control what we can control.* We all know that we *should* have a good posture, but it does not seem to appear too high on our list of priorities. And why should it? Surely it is more important to put food on the table. Of course, it is, which is precisely why many people undertake 'back-breaking' work to support themselves and feed their families.

For those people who engage in hard labour of this nature, furniture removal guys, appliance and furniture delivery guys, builders, gardeners etc. - the fact that the nature of their jobs requires movement is good and they must look after their bodies by learning to do the heavy lifting without damaging their backs and health[82]. I must emphasise nonetheless, that body control and regaining the movement that we had when we were four years old is only going to improve our years of healthy living. Personally, I would like to enjoy the food on my table when I am 80 years old without assistance, wouldn't you?

How many times have you heard the words "Stand up straight!", "Sit up straight!", "Don't slouch!"? That is timeless advice we have probably all heard at one time or another, and I have to say that it is worth taking.

Poor posture is not necessarily only the result of bad habits. There are also some physical reasons for poor posture. These include inflexible muscles that decrease the range of motion of a joint. In other words, muscles can limit how far a joint can move in any direction. For example, if you have overly tight, shortened hip flexor muscles they can pull your upper body forward and disrupt your posture.

Think about all the sitting we do. The muscles on the front of our hips shorten over time, yet when we stand up, we do not walk bent forwards. Why? Because something is pulling us upright. The big muscles of the back are responsible for this, and they will eventually fatigue causing stiffness and pain. I now would like to introduce you to another of our friends, called *Stiff Back*.

To add insult to this injury, weak core muscles encourage slumping, as the body is not able to hold its own weight anymore, which tips your body forward and off balance. Strong lower leg muscles also help keep you steady when you are standing. The positive news is that you can improve your

---

[82] My work is also physical in nature - bending, moving and lifting bodies all day. When I started working, I remember my back paining. And I remember thinking to myself 'How on earth can I have back pain at the age of 24?'. So, I made some physical changes to the rig and started to move more efficiently. I became *work fit* (being fit enough to get through a full workday without pain). The following few chapters portray the tried and tested foundations to becoming *work fit* and having a functional body. *Hint hint.*

posture with a few simple exercises. Before we get into these, lets evaluate whether we have good posture on not.

Medicinal drugs will not correct bad posture. What will correct it is putting your body through a Neural Re-Education protocol and performing many small stretches over a few weeks. Essential to this would also be changing your posture to teach the body its new *normal* posture.

Good posture means:
Chin parallel to the floor
Shoulders level (roll your shoulders up, back, and down to help achieve this)
Neutral spine (no flexing or arching to overemphasize the curve in your lower back)
Arms at your sides with elbows straight and level
Abdominal muscles braced
Hips level
Knees level and pointing straight ahead
Body weight distributed evenly on both feet.
When sitting down, keep your chin parallel to the floor; your shoulders, hips, and knees at even heights; and your knees and feet pointing straight ahead. Do not use a back rest or lumbar support. Ultimately try and sit for the least amount of time that you need to.

Resetting Normal

I often explain to patients that we need to "reset normal"[83] (Concept one: Move how you were designed to move). By this I mean that we need, throughout the day, to counteract these postural mess-ups.

One way to view good posture is to view it as a type of

---

[83] NRE. *Neural Re-Education*. I hope this word is becoming familiar by now.

sport. When you start practicing for it, you will be unfit, it will feel unnatural and you will certainly feel it the next day. Good posture is also classified as a sport in my eyes as you need core muscle activation, some above average[84] flexibility and some spinal proprioception to perform it eloquently.

The three stretches that I show to every one of my patients, and that I do regularly myself (to counteract our 21st century postures) are pectoral stretching, hip flexor stretching and gluteal muscle stretching. (A picture detailing the three essential posture correcting stretches can be found at the end of this chapter.)

Hundreds Club

To compliment these stretches, one of the best NRE tactics you can do to better your posture is called Hundreds Club. Hundreds Club is an exclusive member only club, where the membership is free, and it is open to anyone to join. Okay, so it is not really a club at all. If you think about the 21st century scenario, most of the day we use our hands in front of us. These small movements are called fine motor movements. So, when are we ever using our back muscles for the same small movements? Almost never.

Hundreds Club is one way to counteract this. Basically, you stand on one leg and extend your arms out to either side, while you make 100 small circular rotations (forwards or backwards) with your arms. Imagine you have a pen in each hand, and you are trying to draw 100 tiny circles on the wall behind you. It is a great way to activate all the deep muscles of your neck and upper back, the ones that generally weaken with many hours of sitting.

---

[84] Quite often, whilst I am trying to find a positive or polite way of saying that someone's flexibility is horrible, I describe their flexibility to them as 'above average'. Patients, especially guys, are far too happy about that description.

Of course, I also slouch. You will have the privilege of catching out the teacher occasionally. But when I do slouch, my body immediately reminds me to sit up straight. It becomes instinctive. You too can develop that good *neural* instinct or habit. Perform these three stretches repeatedly throughout your day, every hour to induce a change. Join Hundreds Club twice a day. Remember from the concepts I emphasised; *change is inevitable.* Exaggerate the frequency of the stretches and Hundreds Club for three weeks and you would be well on your way to having developed your 'new normal' posture. It would be like putting yourself through an off-season like any professional athlete would (more on this in the chapter *Recovery, Sleep and Off-seasons*).

Remember this: developing a good habit takes discipline. Maintaining it is the easy part. I perform these stretches two or three times a day now, purely to maintain the 'new normal' posture.

Sitting is the New Smoking

When doctors speak about cancer and smoking, the connection between the two is measured by something called pack-years. A pack-year is a unit for measuring the amount a person has smoked over their life. It is calculated by multiplying the number of packs of cigarettes smoked per day by the number of years the person has smoked. So, one pack a day for one year is one pack-year. One pack a day for five years is five pack-years etc. The quantification of pack-years smoked is important in clinical care, where the degree of tobacco exposure is correlated to be a risk of disease such as lung cancer.

I have come up with a similar quantification tool called sitting-years. A sitting-year is a unit for measuring the amount a person has sat, incorrectly, over their adult life. It is calculated by multiplying the number of days spent sitting (for more than six hours of a workday) by the number of years the person has worked in their job. So, an average of six hours sitting per workday for one year is one sitting-year, five years is five sitting-years etc.

It is a great practical tool to help educate patients on the detriment of prolonged incorrect sitting. The quantification of sitting-years is important in clinical care, where the degree of long-term and incorrect sitting is correlated to be a risk of disc disease, back pain and headaches. Of course this is a gross estimation and is not a direct indicator of these ailments, but the association that I have witnessed between sitting and spine issues, in private practice, is incredible. This is one of the many reasons to take hourly breaks from sitting, to sit properly when you do sit, or to try a standing desk option at work (if possible).

To explain why sitting is so bad and creates such a long-lasting problem to fix I would like to introduce the Overload Theory, that as I understand it, supposes that the body develops muscle where it is needed. If we are sitting for two thirds of our waking hours, sitting muscles will *overload*. Sitting posture develops short hip flexors and shoulder internal rotators.

Since university, I have had the privilege of reading X-rays. I think we take it for granted how astonishing an X-ray is, how we can measure the spine and its curves to a millimetre. The real joy for me is to use this tool to help people.

Clinically, I have observed that 100 out of every 100 X-rays will show degenerative changes in the cervical spine (the neck) when there are degenerative changes at the lumbar spine (the lower back), and vice versa; degenerative changes in the lower back are observable when there are degenerative changes in the neck. This is alarming.

Even more alarming is the fact that one of the areas will often be asymptomatic - it will show no pain whatsoever. That means the neck and lower back are often degenerating at the same rate, and you would not even know it.

Let us look at an example.

December 2016

Phil Dunphy, a 47-year-old male presents to the clinic. He explains he has a lot of family stress due to several different dynamics within the family, and that he injured his lower back jumping on a trampoline.

Patient presents with acute back pain (also a history of low back aches and pains but nothing serious enough to visit a chiropractor) and reports a significant motor vehicle accident 20 years prior.

We ruled out Kummel disease (a variation of avascular necrosis - basically the bone loses its blood supply and begins to die).

Physical examination indicated a low back mechanical strain. The neck however is interesting. On the neurological examination, patient shows absent reflexes C6 left and C7 right. There is dermatomal loss of sensation C5/6/7 on the left.

X-rays were justified and taken. Lumbar spine series shows generalized degenerative changes as expected. The cervical spine series shows complete reverse curvature, and severe disc degeneration with osteophyte formation C5/6/7, indicative of disc degenerative disease at those levels.

The good-to-knows:

ONE. Phil came in with a low back complaint from a trampoline manoeuvre[85]. Without any history of neck pain, his neck shows significant degeneration.

TWO. Pain is a poor indicator of dysfunction and pain often

---

[85] People hurt themselves doing weird things. We see so many patients who hurt themselves during sex. Or descriptions of weird and outrageous acts of desire. Neck pain is common. I have seen throat pain. Lower back pain is common. Strained leg muscles are common. The only case of its nature to date, was presented by a patient who hurt his shoulder trying to have sex whilst attempting a handstand. Not recommended apparently.

is the last symptom to show.

THREE. Could this have been prevented? To some degree, yes. Had he presented to a chiropractor ten to fifteen years before this consultation, lifestyle changes could have been introduced to prevent and slow down the degenerative changes in his spine.

Spine First

We have only one spine. We might as well look after it. The reason why sitting is so bad for you, clinically, is because of what happens to the discs over time.

I cannot tell you how many times I have shown X-rays to patients and they are shocked at the state of their spines because they have never had pain in the area[86].

Why is this? If you look at the spine from the side, the neck and lower back have almost identical curves - they both bend backwards. Now what the 21st century and sitting dominance has done is put excessive forward bending stress on these curves. The discs on the front of the spine take strain and the facet joints wear and tear. Look out for another picture at the end of this chapter, which metaphorically speaking, is what I live for (the picture on the left is a neck x-ray, and the MRI is on the right).

---

[86] Pain is only one symptom. Stiffness or tightness are also symptoms. Remember, it is NOT normal to get a stiff neck, it tells you the body is compensating for something. It is NOT normal to have a stiff lower back. Something is happening, see someone about it.

Slipped Discs

Discs are the cushions between vertebrae, and a disc is simply a water balloon.

I have never seen an intervertebral disc *slip* out of place. Anatomically, the disc is embedded inside a sandwich of bone and ligaments. I have seen this during the dissection of cadavers in 1st and 2nd year Anatomy classes, and this is an accurate description. The notion of a *slipped disc* is therefore a nonsensical term that leads people to think that you can push it back into place. This is certainly not true and creates a big misconception of how you would treat a disc[87].

A disc has only so much life in it. It is literally the same as a cushion on your couch. If you sit on it all the time, it loses its bounce. A disc has an inner gel called the nucleus palposis, and with enough of this stress that we have spoken about above, the gel pushes through the disc.

Once a disc has lost its cushion effect, the disc above it or below it will take double the strain. Theoretically there is now exponentially more strain on the discs above and below, and then the next disc loses its integrity, and so it continues. This type of dysfunction spreads faster than the water leak spread through the Titanic.

If you squeeze a water balloon in your hand, it bulges outwards somewhere, right? That is what happens to a disc. Many years of incorrect postures and poor bending form result in the fluid tracking through the disc slowly. If this process is sudden, then a huge herniation occurs, which in my experience is extremely rare. Most cases are chronic and happen over years, until one day a minuscule incident occurs, such as bending to pick up a cup off a coffee table, and the disc bulges

---

[87] Speaking about misconceptions. Sometimes coming from a foreign land, international jargon is a problem. I had a patient in London who was a barrister (a prominent lawyer). In South Africa, we would use the term lawyer or attorney to describe her vocation. You can imagine her confusion when I asked her how long it took her to learn the art of coffee making (barista).

outwards. Only then do we see symptoms. Symptoms occur because the bulge pushes into the spinal canal or just next to the canal where the nerves exit.

Pins and Needles

To treat a disc, you need to take mechanical strain off it, and over a six-week period, the symptoms will usually ease. Your body will literally absorb the unwanted fluid bulge. The net result after a disc injury is a disc with less cushion ability. The most important reason to maintain normal movement in the pelvis is that this causes less dependence on the spine to take load.

Many patients have a disc surgery without mechanical treatment to restore normal movement. Surgery is either a discectomy, where the surgeon cuts the bulge away, or the surgeon will fuse the segments above and below with metalwork to take away the compression on the disc. This will leave the spine less mobile and ultimately the disc above or below the injured disc will suffer the same consequences.

There is now a potential cascade of events.

ONE. The body is forced to load other structures. It will load the facet joints at the back of the vertebrae, which leads to inflamed joints (arthritis).

TWO. The ligaments in and around the spinal column strain and can eventually ossify over a long period of time.

THREE. Tendons and muscles do more work to keep the spine moving, leading to tension and referred pain.

FOUR. Over years, bones will also change shape and the disc flattens. We see this clearly on X-rays[88].

---

[88] In South Africa, I would often explain to a patient that their disc on X-ray is now *Platteland*. 'Platteland' is an Afrikaans word for the vast flat land situated in the Karoo. I needed to find a replacement word for it when I moved to London, and I came up with *Amsterdam*. It is not as catchy unfortunately.

FIVE. Wolf's Law states that the body will lay bone where it needs support. We notice that these changes often happen on the front of the spine, where we all bend over. Eventually the spine can and will fuse itself as the ligaments and bones unite in ossification.

The good news is that we can prevent this.

All it takes is to start and keep moving. You may need help to get all the joints and muscles moving correctly at first, and that is why there are chiropractors, physiotherapists, sports therapists, and the like. There is method in the midst of all the madness.

The moral of the story is to try conservative decompression first. If I cannot drastically improve a disc patient in six weeks, I refer them directly to the neurosurgeon. We always refer long before that if there is any progressing neurological fallout or severe muscle paralysis or cauda equina whispers[89].

The most important thing to understand here is that we can see signs that a disc is undergoing degenerative changes long before it is ever symptomatic, and if we keep it moving, nutrition to the disc is maintained and you can prevent the damage. By the time you experience *pins and needles*, you are playing catchup with your spine's health (but it is never too late!).

The following chapter speaks into a recommendation that I give to most, if not all, patients. Something that has the power to change your health trajectory on its own.

---

[89] The "whispers" reference is to the film "The Horse Whisperer". Cauda equina syndrome is a condition that occurs when the bundle of nerves below the end of the spinal cord known as the cauda equina is damaged, usually by a centrally herniating disc. The signs and symptoms are a numbness around the anus and groin and loss of bowel or bladder control. These are red flags.

Point to ponder: Are you trying to be more like a bobblehead yet?

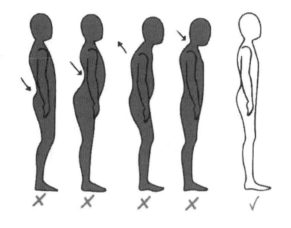

Posture Correction Stretches

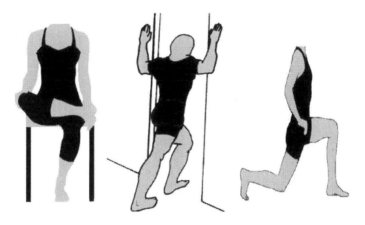

Seated Gluteal Stretch   Doorway Pectoral Stretch   Lunge Hip Flexor Stretch

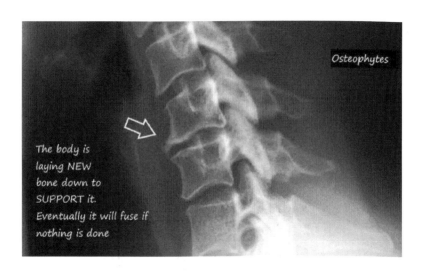

Osteophytes

The body is laying NEW bone down to SUPPORT it. Eventually it will fuse if nothing is done

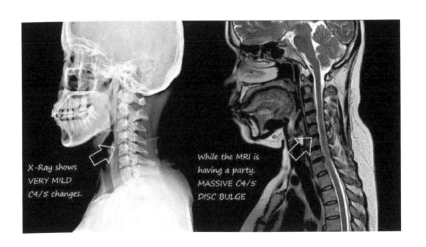

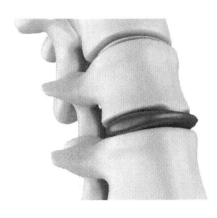

The only way
to PROTECT a
disc is to take

PRESSURE off it
and
SUPPORT it

7 : Zone 2

Jon's medication list includes GP prescribed antidepressant medication. Sertraline Hydrochloride 100mg daily. Three years. Patient attributes his headaches to the medication. Medicine cannot correct mechanics.

Regardless of your fitness level or your affinity (or lack thereof) for exercise, there is always some form of movement you can do to improve and tilt the healing curve in your favour. Clinically, this is my number one recommendation to all my patients. And the recommendation that is often not well publicized, and opposite to what the general media recommends.

This stage of my learning is called: Run slower.

You will see in later chapters that my personal approach to exercising, eating and recovery did not always tilt the healing curve in my favour. Do not make the same mistakes that I did. In terms of running, it is simple - run (mostly) slower to get faster. Run (mostly) slower to avoid niggles. Run (mostly) slower to promote healing. Run (mostly) in Zone 2. We have many discussions about the day-to-day application of Zone 2 later, but for now it is imperative to understand the importance of this kind of exercise.

What is Zone 2?

Zone 2 is a pace you run, cycle, or perform any cardiovascular exercise at. Zone 2 is the intensity that your body exercises in, that puts your body into the *recovery zone.*

Zone 2 also refers to a system of exercise designed to promote recovery, decrease inflammation, decrease stress, and decrease pain by inducing and aiding Neural Re-education (restoring normal movement).

When would you use Zone 2?

Zone 2 is for most running, cycling or endurance exercises.

Is your Zone 2 pace always the same?

No[90].

How do you work out your pace?

The MoveMed equation to work out your Zone 2 pace works out to be the pace or intensity that you can hold 72% or less of your maximum heart rate while exercising.

For me, while running, Zone 2 is a pace that I can run at while holding a heart rate of 143 beats or lower. This is based on the equation below. My maximum heart rate while running, recently, has reached 200 beats per minute.

---

[90] This is the crux of Zone 2 training. The pace is relative to how your body is feeling on the day. I have Zone 2 days when my body feels good and I am fully recovered. We observed that in the previous chapter. Sometimes the pace, for me, will be under five minutes per kilometre. I also have days when the body is knackered and not fully recovered. The pace on those days slows down to six minutes per kilometre. The important thing for fitness is time on your legs, as this builds your neuromusculoskeletal memory base. Refer back to my New York marathon as to just how effective this training is.

Zone 2 = maximum HR for running x 72%

200 x 0.72 = 144

For me, while cycling, Zone 2 is a pace that I can cycle at whilst holding a heart rate of 129 beats or lower.

Zone 2 = maximum HR for cycling x 72%

180 x 0.72 = 129.6

Does it apply to exercises like core, stretching, gym etc.?
No.

While doing Yoga, Pilates or other body weight core exercise, Zone 2 is not applicable. These exercises normally include rest periods where one's heart rate drops drastically. Therefore, my average heart rate for these exercises is always far below Zone 2. Or take a HIIT (high intensity interval training), often my average resting heart for these exercise sessions is above Zone 2.

How do you know what your maximum heart rate is if you are not regularly doing exercise, and how would you work this out?

In keeping this answer as simple as possible, you can use a projected temporary maximum heart rate. There is a simple equation for this, and it can be used to determine your maximum heart rate until you are fit / healthy enough to perform a maximum effort run or cycle.

(Temporary) maximum HR = 225 - your age

HR = 225 – 30 = 195

If you do not have the energy to take your heart rate all the time, and you want to keep it even more simple, how do you describe Zone 2?

Zone 2 is the pace or intensity at which you can perform comfortable exercise, while holding a comfortable conversation with someone. And a bit slower than this pace[91]. Originally Zone 2 was defined as *easy talking* pace. After years of trial and error in my personal fitness, and while working alongside Clinton, we performed unofficial research to get to the golden number of 72%.

This training method is a guide, and a safe way to gauge whether you are training too hard. Importantly, the Zone 2 system is most successful when used in conjunction with keeping track of your resting heart rate. At the risk of sounding repetitive, I would like to emphasise the four main reasons that the Zone 2 training method is essential for a recovery-driven lifestyle.

Recovery (It aids recovery.)
Stress (It decreases stress.)
Inflammation (It decreases inflammation.)
NRE (It aids Neural Re-Education.)

RECOVERY

You can train as much as you want in Zone 2. You will improve your cardiovascular health while recovering from the previous day's workload and stress.

What I have seen with athletes is that their fitness gains are causally related to their quality of recovery. What I have seen with patients is that their response to treatment gains are also causally related to their quality of recovery.

If 80-90% of activities should be in Zone 2, what about the other 15-odd percentage? Spend this time in the Red Zone where there are no rules. You push. You stress your body to a

---

[91] What I often do is I call my friends while I am running. Earphones and microphones are surprisingly functional while doing exercise. My friends on the other end of the line are mostly shocked when, halfway through the hour conversation, they hear a car hooter and realise that I have been running the whole time. Ask my mom, she is often on the other end of the line.

point where it naturally engages super-compensation. Run so fast or do hill work and speed work to the point that you undergo micro-damage. This includes small tears in muscles and tendons, and stretching of ligaments, which may cause inflammation.

Provided you supplement this with enough Zone 2 recovery, good fuel in the form of clean eating, and enough sleep, the body will repair better than before. That is how you get faster, and clinically that is how you heal.

In practice, we stress joints and muscles into ranges of motion they have not been in for a while. We introduce a new and necessary trauma. The key here is adequate recovery. New trauma will heal better than before, and hence restore normal mechanics. This is a vitally important concept in understanding why injuries often get worse before they get better[92].

Here is an example.

September 2019

Don Draper, a 32-year-old male presents to the clinic. His exact words are "I'm not a madman, it feels like my spine is not straight".

Don is currently asymptomatic[93].

---

[92] Concept eight from Chapter five. Things often get worse before they get better. When I make a patient's pain worse for a day or two, it means we have hit the right spots, that is good. More often than not, the pain decreases from day one, this is great. When NOTHING happens, that is a red flag, refer.

[93] He has no pain or symptoms, which tells me that Don is coming in for an assessment. This demonstrates to me that Don is investing in his health by taking the first step of healing; making a quality decision. Be like Don.

We ruled out Scheuermann's disease[94].
X-rays were justified and taken. Don has an S-shaped scoliosis, more than 15 degrees each way. This is significant. Patient responds to NRE protocol and prescribed lifestyle changes.

This is how we explain the NRE protocol to Don: *"The aim of treatment is to slow down the rate at which your scoliosis is getting worse. Treatments will include myofascial release and adjustments. We cause microtrauma by mechanically reducing the curvature in your spine. Provided you help your body recover, it will get stronger in the new position. You will experience pain as your body moves differently initially. As your body loads a joint that it has not used in a while, it causes inflammation which will be experienced as pain. This is necessary to restore normal movement. It is a process. All we ask is that you are patient during this process. I will remind you of this conversation in a few weeks' time".*

During the six-week initial phase, Don experiences bouts of excruciating pain. Painful episodes last two to three days. Don continues with Zone 2 exercise. Over the twelve weeks that follow, his painful episodes and treatment frequency simultaneously diminish. Six-month follow-up and reassessment X-rays show the curvature has improved to 12 degrees each way. Don experiences minimal painful episodes and maintained his Zone 2 exercise. I do not see room for more

---

94 Scheuermann's disease is a condition where you develop an excessively forward rounded back; Quasimodo would have possibly had this, coupled with scoliosis. X-rays of a spine affected by Scheuermann's disease, clearly show the vertebrae becoming forwardly angled over time, and often show Schmorl's nodes too, where the disc herniates into the vertebra itself over time. There is more to what a chiropractor does than simply 'cracking' backs.

improvement in Don's condition as his scoliosis is structural[95], however his prognosis is good in terms of preventing the progression of the curve.

The good-to-knows:

ONE. The difficult part of treating Don was accepting that sometimes you cannot completely cure someone. Sometimes the sheer physics of the spine prevents it, as in Don's case. Sometimes the psychology prevents it, like in the *F-word* chapter towards the end of the book.

TWO. I consider this case a win. Why? Because Don is positive and pro-active in the management of his health. Sometimes, the prevention of things becoming structurally worse, is as good as it gets.

STRESS

"We find ourselves caught in a messed-up world." This is a quote from a sermon Martin Luther King delivered in 1954. Although, some would suggest that people the world over have never been more stressed than they are now in 2020, some would argue that nothing has changed[96]. The next reason for Zone 2 exercise, is its effect on stress.

---

[95] Scoliosis is where the spine is curved when you look straight at it. You get a functional scoliosis, when the spine *appears* to be curved, but the apparent curvature is the result of an irregularity elsewhere in the body. An example is children who carry a heavy schoolbag on the same shoulder for a prolonged time. Another example is different leg lengths. This can, more often than not, be corrected. A structural scoliosis is when the patient's spine actually has a physical curve. The vertebra bones themselves have changed shape. In other words, they have started to become *wedge* shaped as opposed to *rectangular*.

[96] It is funny how we always compare situations. Someone will say "you don't know what stress is". Never take away the relativity of someone's situation. Everyone has their own hurts and worries. If history has taught us anything it is that the world needs a lot more love, but we just cannot seem to get it right. Stand against the haters, show love.

Too much stress - financial, emotional, chemical, you name it - breaks down the body. It prevents healing. It prevents rebuilding. It prevents recovery. For a third of our lives, give or take eight hours a day, most of us are in a work environment. This is a stressful environment. Therefore, it is safe to say that for a third of our lives, we are in a stressed state.

The body releases Cortisol when it is stressed[97]. Cortisol is a hormone and is catabolic in nature; that means it breaks down the body. The same happens with emotional stress in the home environment, whether one feels unsafe in one's home or one is struggling through challenging personal relationships, Cortisol is released. For some of us, just seeing two blue ticks next to the WhatsApp message we sent and anxiously waiting for a reply can cause a release of Cortisol. Stress is relative.

Even the food we eat can cause chemical stress, causing a leaky gut[98] and again breaking down the body as opposed to rebuilding and healing it. And again, more Cortisol is released.

For many of us in high-paced, high stakes, high-pressure day jobs, we are in a stressed or catabolic state internally. This tilts our healing and recovery seesaw in favour of destruction. Logically, it makes sense to add a stimulus that antagonises that ratio, that does something to tilt the seesaw back into a healing dominance. I propose that that something is Zone 2 exercise.

---

[97] A quick check in. Cortisol is the hormone that produces the fight or flight reaction to any stress. Great when you run into a wild animal in Africa, not great when you are sitting at your desk and predominantly stationary.

[98] More on this in the diet chapter later. But an unhealthy gut lining may allow partially digested food, toxins, and bugs to penetrate the tissues beneath it. This may trigger inflammation. We all have some degree of leaky gut, as this barrier is not completely impenetrable. Some of us may have a genetic predisposition and may be more sensitive to changes in the digestive system. Modern lifestyles may be the main driver of gut inflammation. Diets that are low in fibre and high in sugar and saturated fats, may start the process. Heavy alcohol, of course, has the same effect. And so does stress.

Clinically, Zone 2 exercise stops the Cortisol cycle and releases chemicals like endorphins and cannabinoids. Clinically, this helps to create a healing environment. Too much Red Zone exercise will add stress to our bodies, drastically affecting our quality of recovery, (if there is any).

If you are incredibly stressed at work and want to exercise to decompress that stress, Zone 2 is the way to go. Mental and emotional stress, coupled with physical stress (Red Zone exercise), are an overload.

If you want to know how much is *too much*, this is a relative term. Learn to listen to your body, or how to take your resting heart rate at the very least[99].

INFLAMMATION

The third reason to incorporate Zone 2 running is its effect on inflammation.

The saying "too much of a good thing" applies to much of life. Especially to inflammation. People think inflammation needs to be eradicated constantly and completely. This is fake news. Inflammation plays an essential role in healing and injury repair to keep your body safe and healthy. Inflammation, and pain, tell you that something is wrong. When we have an acute injury or microbe incursion, inflammation is the natural and normal protective response from our bodies; one that is essential for our survival.

Without inflammation, we could die from a bruised muscle or a common cold, but too much of a good thing can be bad for you, and when inflammation is chronic, it becomes disease-causing rather than life-saving. In excess, inflammation leads to scar tissue and mechanical

---

[99] Spoiler for a later chapter called *'Wear your heart on your sleeve'* where we detail the simplest way of tracking how your body is recovering.

restriction[100].

Here is one example. Most doctors are likely to advise that one should avoid running once diagnosed with tendonitis. I have found that strictly staying in Zone 2 will not further damage the tendon, in fact, it is reparative. However, it is vitally important not to go into the Red Zone at all when you are injured or nursing a niggle[101]. Overuse injuries (the name gives it away), get worse with overuse. Overuse occurs when the healing seesaw tilts in favour of damage as opposed to healing. Zone 2 puts that equation back in our favour.

The main reason to avoid zone 3[102] exercise is that in that zone, the body does not allow inflammation to cease. On the flip side, I would go as far to say that zone 3 exercise causes the most overuse injuries. The constant hammering and bashing away at your cartilage will induce inflammation, and if that inflammation is not allowed to cease naturally, a cascade of reactions occur, like protective muscle spasms and ligament strains. It is literally the definition of overuse injuries: too much inflammation, too little recovery. Compare this with Zone 2, where the impact is low enough to promote

---

[100] Heck, inflammation even causes things like cholesterol to stick to heart walls! One painful and inflamed joint in your spine can leave you walking into the practice like Smeagol. Inception footnote (footnote within a footnote): J. R. R. Tolkien's iconic Lord of the Rings character, Smeagol (or Gollum) who moves about on all four limbs. The body sometimes does this to avoid putting pressure through the inflamed joint. A more basic example is an involuntary limp from a twisted ankle.

[101] During any initial phase of treatment, stay ONLY in Zone 2 if you are exercising. You are playing with fire if you go into red zones while undergoing treatment. In my mind this seems as if I am stating the obvious, but I have found that most patients have not been told this. Look out for Phoebe Buffay's case later in *Recovery, Sleep and Off-seasons*.

[102] Spoiler for later but Zone 3 is from the five zone models of exercise. In my two-zone model, Zone 3 would simply be the pace or intensity that is marginally faster than your Zone 2 effort. Too fast to recover. Too slow to get faster. Where most runners spend most of their time, and why runners commonly get injured. My most humble opinion.

healing, blood flow and adaptation.

NEURAL RE-EDUCATION

The fourth and most important reason for Zone 2 exercise is its effect on the brain. It is a vital part of restoring movement because we must teach the body how to move normally again.

Sometimes it is necessary to go backward to go forward.

When injuries occur, we need to re-educate the body to move in the way it was designed to move[103]. It has been mentioned a few times in this book that any old trauma or injury will lead to abnormal movement patterns, and if not corrected within six weeks of the injury, those abnormal movement patterns will add extra stress onto your musculoskeletal system. It will put you at risk of overuse or repetitive strain injuries in the future.

This is one of the most important things I do for a living - this physiological act of re-educating the body regarding the way it was designed to function.

Joints lock up or become heavily restricted once they have been subjected to a trauma like whiplash, a fall, or years of low-grade trauma from poor posture. When a joint is bruised, inflammation will heal it. However, without movement re-education, scar tissue forms in an abnormal fashion, restricting movement until it is broken down and remodelled. This is the basic premise for rehabilitation.

---

[103] Concept one from Chapter five. *Move how you were designed to move.* More efficient movement decreases stress on the body, further helping the health seesaw tilt in the favour of healing.

A muscle's function is to move a joint or to protect it. An inflamed or strained joint will cause muscle spasm to prevent further injury. The body is brilliant in that way, but a spasm for more than three days becomes problematic because that is when scar tissue starts forming. Joints and muscles that have not been re-educated after an injury will remain restricted.

I see this daily in X-ray studies. We see areas of calcification on X-rays, and what I have deduced is that calcification only happens and can only be seen on X-rays at areas where we can clearly feel there is no movement.

One example can be seen on my own X-rays.

Between the base of my skull and the first neck vertebrae, there is clear calcification happening in the atlantooccipital ligament, the one that surrounds the vertebral artery. How did that happen? Take your pick from the three times I have been hit by a car whilst I was cycling. Looking back, the neck whiplash injuries were never treated mechanically, only with anti-inflammatory medication. I had chronic headaches until I was assessed and treated mechanically. Interesting.

Here is another example.

I describe this to my patients as *white worms*. On the front view of the neck X-ray, we very often see calcification of the vertebral arteries where they run through the vertebra. In other words, we see an outline of what looks like a worm crawling through the neck. This is visible only in areas where we can clearly feel there is no movement. We cannot reverse this calcification, but we can stop it in its tracks, which is a positive prognosis.

So, clinically, when we mobilize immobile joints, release tight muscles, and get a patient moving in a safe exercise zone - Zone 2 - we can eventually restore normal movement. Zone 2 exercise maintains that movement.

From an injury prevention perspective, it is the same thing. We educate the body to move even more efficiently, decrease the wear and tear coefficient of exercise, and ultimately reduce the risk of injury dramatically.

From a sports performance perspective, when you are into the red and your body is shutting down during a race, it is this neuromusculoskeletal memory that kicks in. It is this memory that maintains your form. An efficient form for any athlete means optimal power, no energy loss, and ultimately, speed.

The Power of Neural Re-Education

This is what happens when you put a *healthy* person through a NRE protocol.

Nick Bester is a professional running coach. His testimony regarding the NRE protocol and sports performance is one that I hold in high regard. Nick is professional in every sense of the word, and I was lucky enough to *witness his fitness* first-hand in October 2020 as he attempted to break his marathon time, three months after we began his NRE protocol.

Here are Nick's words, verbatim:

In 2020 I became a full-time running coach. I have been running competitively for seven years and every year I have been able to improve. However, I am now at that stage where the only gains are marginal ones, and these are hard to come by. Any small improvement to my training, or my recovery, is now considered gold.

Cuan reached out to me and said that he had something to offer me. Something that he believed would "make me run faster". Now I was all ears. We initially discussed what my training at the time looked like. We both realised there were some areas that I was neglecting in my training (proprioception exercises, as an example, and the need for more "real" recovery runs that Cuan referred to as Zone 2). This meant there was room for improvement. On top of that, I had run over 25,000 kilometres over the past seven years and I had neglected joint mobility, joint stability and joint control as part of my physical therapy.

Having previously never worked with any chiropractors (I

continue to see physiotherapists in conjunction with Cuan), I never realised just how important true joint mobility was or how the body can develop incorrect movement patterns. In my case these were from years of working and sitting behind a desk in finance and neglecting some basic forms of recovery, all while consistently running over 100km per week.

Cuan explained the benefits of what his Neural Re-Education (NRE) protocol would bring to a marathon runner like myself. He felt that six weeks was the bare minimum we needed to see a physiological change. After discussing these things in depth, I was up for the challenge.

During the initial consultation we found that I had a significant pelvic rotation (resulting in a short right leg), coupled with numerous areas of joint restriction (the joints had forgotten how to move). Every treatment would involve full body muscle trigger point release, stretching and of course the adjustments. He gave me rehabilitation exercises to add to my existing home body weight exercise routines which consisted of proprioception, flexibility and core activations.

At first Cuan would find a similar pattern of restrictions. This was until around the fourth week when Cuan said it felt like his adjustments were "holding" (this meant they had not locked up or restricted themselves between treatments). This was the first sign of physiological changes (of changing the nerve and muscle memory). From here it only improved.

Three weeks after the NRE protocol, we decided to put the body to the test. I would attempt to try run my fastest 5km. I was now seeing Cuan once a week. My previous 5km personal best was 15:20 and this would be difficult to beat as I would attempt to run this race alone. Cuan came to watch, and I managed to finish in 15:16. This was incredible, especially considering that the week building up to the race was one of the hottest weeks in UK's history and my body was drained.

Six weeks after the 5km attempt, while still seeing Cuan weekly, I would attempt to run my fastest Marathon. My previous best was 2.29,50 at the Berlin Marathon in 2019. I was scheduled to race the 2020 London Marathon, however Covid 19 guidelines meant that I would have to run a 'virtual' marathon. Cuan offered to be the "lead bicycle" as a witness to the officiality of the attempt. On that October day at Battersea Park, we were treated to 8-degree temperatures, gale force wind and torrential rain, and somehow, I managed another personal best. 2.28,35. Unbelievable.

There are many variables to why I ran a personal best that day, however it is undeniable the benefit I got from Cuan's NRE protocol. Even if I did not manage to break my personal best, the truth is that I was not injured, I was recovering better, and I could feel that I was running more efficiently. In my business, efficiency means less injury, less injury means consistent marginal gains and consistent gains mean getting better, faster and stronger. The future looks bright.

As a running coach, I recommend this protocol highly and I have already seen the benefits to some of my runners who have worked with him. Not only have I made a good friend in Cuan, but I cannot thank him enough for making me embark on this journey with him. What started off as a six week "project" has now become a weekly occurrence and long may it continue.

We took a picture together, in the freezing cold rain, in Battersea Park, moments after he ran his fastest marathon to date.

The following chapters unpack *how* we can alter, change, and ultimately hold a good posture. These speak to the three pillars of MoveMed - Core, Flexibility and Proprioception.

Point to ponder: Have you been running too fast and too often your entire life, without knowing it?

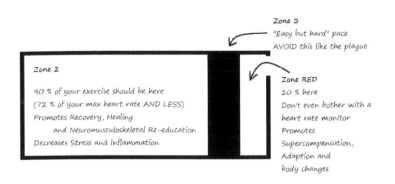

Zone 3
"Easy but hard" pace
AVOID this like the plague

Zone 2

90 % of your exercise should be here
(72 % of your max heart rate AND LESS)
Promotes Recovery, Healing
       and Neuromusculoskeletal Re-education
Decreases Stress and Inflammation

Zone RED
10 % here
Don't even bother with a
heart rate monitor
Promotes
Supercompensation,
Adaption and
body changes

155

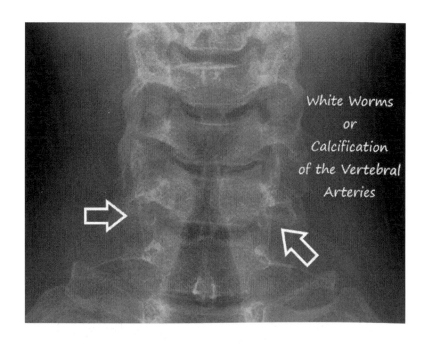

White Worms
or
Calcification
of the Vertebral
Arteries

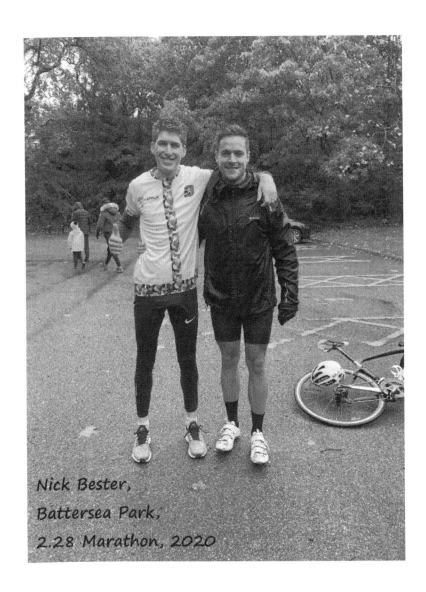

Nick Bester,
Battersea Park,
2.28 Marathon, 2020

8 : Core

Jon's significant adult trauma: Car accident, aged 23, head on, hit a stationary car from behind while travelling >100km/h. Whiplash treated with a neck brace for 3 months. *A neck brace for that long probably did more damage than the car accident did. Assume that normal movement was never restored.*

A current popular buzz word in the health and fitness industry is *"Core"*. However, this word is prolifically misunderstood.

When most people think about core strength, they think about an abdominal six-pack. While it looks good, (to some), this defined outer layer of abdominal musculature is quite the opposite to a strong core. In fact, overtraining abdominal muscles can set you up for injuries and cut athletic prowess.

Abdominal muscles bend the spine forwards (into flexion), and if you remember the last chapter, we are trying to avoid this spinal flexion as it is dominating our modern-era postures. The core includes the muscles of the pelvic floor (ladies will know about these), all the muscles around your waist (the abs, obliques, lats, erectors), and the hip flexors, to name a few. The combination of all these muscles working in good order creates a strong and a stable base to control movements, transfer energy, and prevent injury.

With this in mind, it is important to understand that your core can fall asleep. That is to say that our core muscle activation and core muscle strength are consistently weakening because we all use back rests, chairs, and seatbelts. Remember from the concepts: *If you do not use it, you lose it?* The more we use artificial support for our spines, the less our core is activated. In turn, this has a negative neuromusculoskeletal memory effect on the motor cortex in our brain, and the body stops activating the core before movement[104].

Basic engineering concepts and structural designs, such as those used in the design of the Egyptian pyramids, for example, teach us that you need to have a strong base. Look at the leaning tower of Pisa. If the base is weak, the effects are evident. These days I see too many leaning towers; overweight stomachs pulling the spine forward into flexion.

The most important benefits of a strong core are improved balance and stability, which results in a supported spine during movement. This directly decreases spinal degeneration. It is that simple.

I like to think of the core as the body's base. A weak link in the body can be likened to a poor foundation of a building. Once force is applied to that building in a certain way it will collapse due to the weakness within its structure. The exact

---

[104] You bend down to pick up a heavy load of washing. The first muscles to fire should be your core muscles, as these support your spine during bending. Instead, since our lifestyles tend to nurture a weak, or worse, an asleep core, we lose that initial activation. The next thing to happen a few years later whilst you are bending down to move the couch to retrieve your TV remote, is that your spine acts alone without core support, and BOOM, your disc explodes. The end of Chapter 14 shows an exploded L4/5 disc on an MRI, look out for it.

same mechanical principle applies to the body and associated injury. A common injury related to poor core strength is low back pain. If an individual has imbalances throughout the core musculature, or if these muscles lack strength, an excessive load can be placed on the low back - often causing discomfort or injury.

Think of your core muscles as the sturdy central link in a chain that connects your upper body and your lower body. The core is a corset of muscles designed to support the vertebrae, inter-segmentally, between each vertebra, during any movement. The core also includes the pelvic floor musculature, and the key here is that the core is meant to activate first, and subconsciously, before movement of your arms or legs. Whether you are hitting a tennis ball or mopping the floor, the necessary motions either originate in your core, or move through it.

No matter where movement starts, it ripples upward and downward through your spine. The weak or inflexible core muscles can therefore drastically affect how well your arms and legs function. That, in turn, simply means that your body will start using power muscles to do posture work, and this decreases the amount of power available to move you. Properly building up your core elevates your power. A strong core also enhances balance and stability. Thus, it can help prevent falls and injuries during sports or other activities. In fact, a strong, flexible core is the cornerstone of almost everything we do.

Gym Machines

The fitness industry and most famous body builders teach us to utilise single muscle movements. Consider, for example, gym machines and free weights. Have you ever wondered why a machine was introduced into a gym? It is to decrease the number of hired staff. Lower overheads mean greater returns.

This is business 101[105]. What a gym apparatus teaches the body is to use one muscle at a time, usually while the core is not active as you are sitting on the machine. The body eventually starts using isolated muscles to perform the activities of daily living, and I have seen many examples of how this leads to an injury.

Take the hamstring muscles as one example (the massive group of muscles behind your thigh). A beautifully powerful muscle that pulls your leg backwards while running, helps to extend your back and slows your body down after jumping off a ledge. The muscle is designed to 'fire' only when other muscle groups such as the core have already supported the spine etc. If you use the 'hamstring machine' at the gym, that teaches the hamstring to 'fire' on its own. And one day you find yourself playing a social game of football or touch rugby, and whilst changing direction, your hamstrings 'fire' on their own or before they are meant to, and boom. *Torn.*

Another example. Certain gym machines could teach the core 'not to fire'. The lower back is vulnerable to injury if the core is not supporting it. One day you are lifting a mildly heavy box to place on top of a shelf at home and (because there was no support for it), boom. *Strained lower back.*

To avoid these, we should rather prioritise the spine. We should focus on functional and body weight movement. This is called the first philosophy of movement, which means that when we focus on a movement the body will recruit the muscles needed to perform that movement. One example is a squat, or a downward dog pose. The body will use the muscles needed to hold the posture or perform the movement. These

---

[105] This trend must have started in greater Europe or the USA where labour is expensive. If you want a quick reason to be grateful where you are, the daily wage for a domestic helper in South Africa is around £6 or $7 per day. A large majority of households live off that. Even more scary, a large portion of the world's population live under $1 per day. Which means earning $7 per day as a domestic helper is considered by many as a good wage, even though it is most certainly not.

are examples of core strengthening.

The Health Lift

As I said earlier, I completed the level one CrossFit coaches' course in 2013 where I learnt comprehensively about functional movements and the history of Olympic weightlifting. It was at this course that we were taught that the deadlift was once called the health lift[106]. When performed correctly, the deadlift is the ultimate weighted movement. The name change came when gym bunnies started lifting too much weight too soon, (and generally with horrible form), and discs started to explode. By that I mean that there was an increased incidence of low back pain and slipped discs.

When performed correctly, the deadlift activates almost every muscle in the body but allows muscles to perform their true function. But this occurs only when the lift is performed correctly. I cannot stress that point enough.

Let me explain. The mistake most people make in the gym is that their weight or centre of gravity is through their toes, as opposed to through their heels.

Here is the *incorrect* deadlift scenario. Your weight goes through your toes. This activates the front (anterior) chain of muscles (shin muscles, quads and the hip flexors) and ultimately activates the deep spinal flexors that bend the spine forwards. Alarm bells start ringing - remember how this kind of spinal flexion increases disc pressure?

Here is the *correct* deadlift scenario. Your weight goes through your heels. This activates the back (posterior) chain of

---

[106] Which turned out to be fake news. The 'Health Lift' was simple, basically: 'Pile heavy objects onto a machine, and then lift it. Workout completed, fitness and health improved'. Turns out that the 'Health Lift' evolved into what we know as a 'deadlift', The object is lifted as a 'dead weight' with no momentum or leverage used to aid the lift. The deadlift is arguably the best all-around lift for full-body strength and muscle development. Ask Arnie.

muscles. Activation is your calves, hamstrings, glutes and ultimately the lower back extensors (quadratus lumborum or QL) and your lats. The spine is pulled backwards (into extension), and this is good. The lower back is meant to be bending backwards, and now the spine is the priority.

The easiest way to fix to your gym lifting form is to lift your toes off the ground, inside your shoes. Try it right now. Try a bodyweight squat. Then try it again with your toes off the ground. It is a game changer.

Low Back Pain

Have you ever had low back pain? If not, I am sure you have heard people complain that their backs are sore. Nobody takes low back pain seriously until they have experienced it. Unlike a sprained ankle joint, where you can limp and avoid loading it, a sprained facet joint in your low back is excruciating. You cannot limp to avoid it as it is a central weight-bearing joint. The body collapses and you hear people say things like "I literally cannot move" or "Please help me get up".

This debilitating problem, which affects around one-third of the UK adult population each year, may be prevented by exercises that promote well-balanced, and more importantly, active core muscles. When back pain occurs, a protocol of core exercises is often prescribed to relieve it, coupled with medications, physical therapy, or other treatments if necessary. Why not rather prevent it?

Here are some scary statistics.

It is estimated that up to eight in every ten people in the UK are affected by back pain at some point in their lives. That is correct - eight out of ten. That is the reality. I see this, in my practice, during routine case histories. I would say that nine out of ten patients verbalize the fact that they have experienced back pain.

Chronic pain affects between one-third and one-half of the population of the UK, that translates to just under 28 million adults[107]. I believe this number is as high is 80 or 90 percent, as pain is often disguised as a tight back, or a tired one. We forget that these are also symptoms of lower back dysfunction.

Back pain is the largest single cause of disability in the world, in the UK, (and in South Africa the last time I checked). It is the most common cause of job-related disability and a leading contributor to missed workdays.

What that looks like in day-to-day living if you are a boss, is that the biggest excuse for employees to miss work would be back pain. Referrals for spinal surgery are also increasing year-on-year, and a growing number of patients are waiting longer than 18 weeks between referral and treatment. I would rather recommend that said patients consult an allied health professional, where the maximum wait is one week[108]. At least attempt conservative treatment before surgery (unless red flags are present of course). This seems like the logical answer, although not the one often chosen by patients[109].

---

[107] This is based on data from available published studies at the time of writing this book. There are, most likely, more recent epidemiological studies available as you are reading this. I would bet my left pinky toe that the incidence is only increasing.

[108] The Allied Health Professions comprise of 14 distinct occupations including: art therapists, dietitians, drama therapists, music therapists, occupational therapists, operating department practitioners, orthoptists, osteopaths and chiropractors, paramedics, physiotherapists, podiatrists, prosthetists and orthotists, diagnostic and therapeutic radiographers, and speech and language therapists.

[109] Remember, my brother is an orthopaedic surgeon. I refer to surgeons for their opinion and management all the time. They are one of the most essential tiers of medicine. Regarding treatment, sometimes the problem is brought on by the patient themselves. Patients will tell me 'Dr (redacted) said he can perform a spinal fusion surgery next week' or 'Dr (redacted) always operates too quickly'. And I am always thinking 'Okay, so you walked into a surgeon's consultation room, consciously, and you're surprised that they offered you surgery?' No real point here and no one to blame, merely some of my findings that may save you a surgery one day.

Low back pain is the second most common condition for which people see a GP. Again, take some time to digest that; it means that apart from the common flu and sore throats, low back pain is the most common condition that a GP sees. Now a GP can offer only temporary relief in the form of pain medication or anti-inflammatory medication, besides which, in my experience, the chances of your pain coming back after medication alone are extremely high.

Where I think we should be focusing is prevention. The single biggest and well-documented risk for low back pain is lack of exercise. From my experience I would agree - lack of exercise and prolonged stationary postures are common denominators to patients I have seen with chronic back pain.

Balance and Stability

Your core helps to stabilize your body, which allows you to move in any direction, even on uneven terrain, or to stand in one spot without losing your balance (a function known as Proprioception, on which there is an entire chapter later). This, in turn, decreases your risk of falling.

As previously mentioned, a weak core contributes to slouching and communicating insecurity or shyness, while good posture projects confidence. More importantly, it decreases wear and tear on the spine and allows you to breathe deeper. Good posture helps you gain the full benefits and optimal performance from exercise.

A Weak Core

As we grow older, we develop degenerative changes in the spine. It is inevitable. The structures of the bones and cartilage are subject to wear and tear. Something we need to grasp is that we can completely control and eliminate degenerative symptoms with the appropriate core exercises. Having strong and stable postural muscles helps suspend the bones and other structures, allowing them to move better. Scoliosis can also often be managed with the correct postural exercises and mobilization treatments[110].

Here is an example.

April 2017

Barney Stinson, a 32-year-old male patient presented to the clinic. He describes an incident where he was suiting up for his third date of the week, bent forward to put his socks on and injured his back.

Barney is now experiencing severe and debilitating low back pain that is aggravated with bearing down[111]. Pain is described as a numbing tingle burn that extends down the back of the leg, behind the knee and under the foot.

We ruled out Ehlers-Danlos Syndrome (a rare genetic condition causing you to have extremely hypermobile joints. Sounds like a helpful side effect to have - it is not.)

Barney was diagnosed with a disc bulge between the fourth and fifth lumbar segments. He opted to accept our recommendation for conservative treatment instead of an operation. The most significant risk factor for Barney was a lack of core strength. Instead of trying to meet ladies, it would

---

[110] Scoliosis means that if you look straight at the spine from the front or back, there are visible bends in it. This is abnormal. Looking at the spine from the side, the chest forward curve is called kyphosis and the neck and lower back backward curves are called lordosis. These are normal.

[111] Bearing down can only be explained as trying to control a loud flatus. You try increase the pressure inside of you. Medically, this is known as the Valsalva Maneuver, a technique that is one of the most common ways to slightly increase intraspinal pressure. Thus, it may indicate impingement on a nerve by an intervertebral disc or other part of the anatomy.

have benefitted him to do some exercise.

The good-to-knows:

ONE. I describe these as my bread-and-butter patients. By that, I mean that they are the reason, if I ate bread, that I would be able to put bread and butter on the table. It is concerning how often we see this.

TWO. Fast forward six weeks, and Barney is now fully mobile, and his pain is negligible. Prognosis is good.

The reality is that most disc patients I see are aged between 30 and 40. This is noticeably young. The other reality is that most of these cases would be avoidable had the patient been educated about basic core strengthening exercises and used said advice.

Core Exercise

A core-activation program relies less on mindless repetition of exercises and more importantly on awareness. You need to know exactly *how* to activate your core. People with good core strength learn to identify and activate these muscles. Learning to activate the core requires concentration, but it leads to you being more in tune with your body[112].

There is no one method of core activation that works for everyone. Some people prefer classes (although it is easy to become lazy with the repetitions and not fully understand the targeted muscle groups). Others use Pilates or Yoga, (both of which I highly recommend), to discover where their core is.

It sometimes takes a lot of patience for you to 'find' your

---

[112] First time going to a Pilates class is always an eye-opening experience. The instructor gives verbal cues to help you initiate the right muscle activation. For women, the cue is *stopping a wee* or *suck water up and through your vaginal canal.* Yes guys, this is possible. For guys, they explain if *you're standing, lift your testicles up and off the floor.* And yes ladies, this is also possible.

core, but once you do, it can be engaged and easily activated (and on demand), during any activity - including walking, driving, and sitting. When you start with core activation exercises, begin with awareness and control. Athletes can further challenge their stability with more complex movements that can be guided by personal trainers or other fitness specialists. YouTube is a great source of core activation videos, but make sure you watch the correct ones. My YouTube channel has a few safe starter videos you may want to try[113].

Daily practice of core activations can lead to healthier movement patterns that allow for increased mobility and independence throughout the course of your whole life.

Yoga vs Pilates

I am often asked, professionally, which is better? I can honestly say that both are highly effective for core activation. My advice would be to find a class that is convenient and give it a try. Try and find an instructor that you are comfortable with and attend consistently, because they will be able to cater to your fitness level and accommodate any injuries or niggles you might have. Also, invite your friends and family to join you, as I am sure you now know the importance of core for your spine's health.

Pregnancy and Core

It is incredibly important to keep some core activation exercises going during pregnancy. A particularly good friend

---

[113] Simply google my name and surname. It seems that being the only 'Dr Cuan Coetzee' in the world comes in pretty handy for this kind of thing.

of mine, Dr Spring[114], educated me once on pregnancy advice regarding core strength. To summarize, she taught me that generally during pregnancy, one can continue with the intensity of exercise one's body has become accustomed to before becoming pregnant. However, adding a new type of exercise intensity to your pregnant body may only add more stress to the system.

In practice, I have seen that pregnant patients thrive on core activity exercises and Zone 2 intensity exercise. There is a whole lot on this later, but Zone 2 exercise does not induce a stress response in the body, and that is as good as gold.

Regardless of natural or caesarean births, a mother can start core activations six weeks after giving birth. If the scar or wound needs more time than this to heal, or if healing is delayed because a certain older sibling has jumped onto mummy's post-birth belly and tenderised the caesarean cut further, this is fairly normal. When a mother is feeling ready and able to exercise, it is essential to remind the body how the core is meant to activate as the core was being stretched for around 40 weeks during the gestation period. Another reason to do this, is that a new mother often has a poor posture as she naturally undergoes excessive bending and forward slouching in caring for and feeding (breast and bottle) her baby.

Here is one of my pregnant patients.

July 2017

Carrie Bradshaw, a 27-year-old female patient presents to the clinic. She describes an incident involving a rec room and

---

[114] Dr Robyn Spring, a specialist gynaecologist, running enthusiast, loving wife and mother. She taught me everything I know about pregnancy and how to treat new moms. She also taught me what NOT to say to new moms, like: *You're breastfeeding, right?* Or *You are going to vaccinate, right?* Or *My little one slept 12 hours last night.*

a ping pong table and is now 30 weeks pregnant.

Patient describes low back pain with a dull ache extending down her whole leg. She is unable to take medication due to the pregnancy.

We ruled out osteitis deformans (also known as Paget's disease), during which, as the name suggests, the bone (osteo) becomes inflamed (itis) and deformed (deformans).

Carrie's diagnosis is piriformis muscle dysfunction[115], which is frequently secondary to the body's need to support itself[116].

Myofascial release with needles and chiropractic adjustments does the trick, but more essential for Carrie were core activation exercises.

The good-to-knows:

ONE. Carrie gave natural birth at 40 weeks to a healthy baby girl.

TWO. Six weeks after the birth she came in for an assessment as discussed. This six-week post birth session is crucial to begin Neural Re-Education of her new pelvis. We say *new* pelvis because her pelvis underwent 40 weeks of change due to the pregnancy hormones involved in relaxing the ligaments. Now the body starts *tightening up* after birth. 'Tightening up' is complicated by holding and feeding a baby

---

[115] The piriformis is one of the deep muscles in your buttocks. The sciatic nerve, the massive nerve that supplies the entire leg, literally runs through this muscle. If it goes into spasm, the patient presents with numbness, tingles, burning, electrical or shooting pain, that can run down the leg and into the foot. It is especially important to diagnose as it mimics a disc injury, yet much easier and quicker to fix. Knowing this may save you heaps of money, time or surgeries.

[116] Relaxin is a hormone produced by the ovary and the placenta during pregnancy. It basically relaxes the ligaments in the pelvis in preparation for childbirth. Great for allowing the mom to try push out the baby. Not great for your mechanics. Remember that the pelvis is a large weight bearing structure. It now becomes unstable with the relaxing ligaments. And the mother's weight increases thanks to the baby. The body's only way to support itself is with muscle spasm. That is one of the many reasons why, during pregnancy most women hate the third trimester.

and leads to abnormal movement patterns.

THREE. Good advice for new moms is to have an assessment after six weeks or once all scars involved are healed and exercise can begin again.

Pregnancy and Exercise

I value Dr Robyn Spring's advice to new mothers because she has an appreciation for the unique personal journey of each new mother and her baby. On top of this, she is a mother herself and had endometriosis, which was part of the reason for her battling to fall pregnant, while her pregnancy itself was complicated by abnormal hormone levels and later on by preeclampsia. Completing the pregnancy alone was a miracle, but it was her journey back to health and fitness that impressed me the most and from where I have gained much inspiration. In my opinion she is the most qualified person to give advice. I asked her to write a piece for the book and this is what she came up with.

While every woman's circumstances are different and every pregnancy is different, there is no doubt that regular exercise in an uncomplicated pregnancy is beneficial. From improving cardiovascular fitness and psychological wellbeing to reducing the risks associated with a sedentary lifestyle, it is an all-round win.

Without a doubt exercise is safe in pregnancy. It reduces the risk of excessive weight gain, gestational diabetes, preeclampsia, macrosomia (big baby), post-partum water retention, incontinence and depression. Exercise also plays a role in stabilising the pelvic girdle, which can become threatened in pregnancy, thereby reducing pain. and neuralgia[117].

There are, of course, risks attached to exercise - trauma, hyperthermia, a reduction in blood flow through the placenta which can lead to impaired growth of the baby; so, one must be cautious and careful in your choices. One should avoid contact sports and those that involve a lot of jumping.

Because of the effects of progesterone softening ligaments and tendons, one has to be careful with stretching exercises, and these should rather be done in a controlled environment. While yoga is absolutely fine, hot yoga should be avoided because of those hyperthermia risks. One must take care with heavy weightlifting and should also not lie flat on one's back in late pregnancy, as that can reduce blood pressure, making one dizzy and nauseous. Scuba diving, bungee jumping and sky diving should all rather be delayed until one is no longer pregnant!

A general guideline is that during exercise one should always use your heart rate monitor and stay within Zone 2 for cardiovascular exercise.

When should one stop exercising when you are pregnant? If there is any bleeding or leakage of waters, one should report immediately to the hospital. If contractions start, or if one becomes short of breath, dizzy or faint and has any chest pain one should stop immediately and rest, reporting to the hospital if these symptoms do not settle. If there are any issues with balance, one should rather avoid exercise.

Obviously there are also situations when one should not exercise at all, some pre-existing medical conditions and some obstetric complications; therefore one should always have a frank discussion with your doctor about what exercise one

---

[117] *Neura* meaning nerve and *algia* meaning pain. This is a stabbing, burning, tingling, numbing and often severe pain due to an irritated or damaged nerve. The nerve may be anywhere in the body. We spoke about the piriformis muscle causing nerve irritation to the sciatic nerve earlier. This is a prime example of pregnancy related neuralgia.

intends doing and get a clearance from him/her.

(My general rule of thumb - do not try to become a marathon runner if you are not already one. If you are already exercising prior to pregnancy, try to maintain that regime, sticking to the rules of engagement. If you do not exercise, but want to start something, start with some walking or swimming, sticking to the general rules.)

Point to ponder: Is your core on its way to being as strong as a pyramid's?

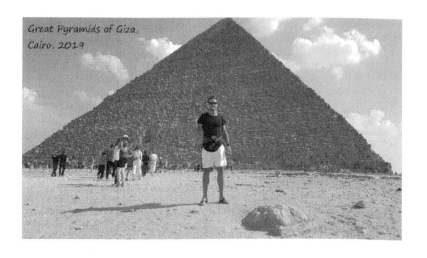

Great Pyramids of Giza,
Cairo, 2019

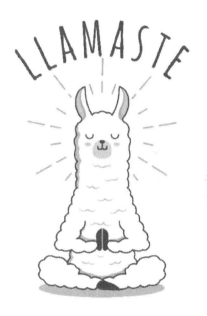

9 : Flexibility

Jon recalls a fall off his bicycle aged 17.
Unconscious for 3 minutes. CT scans at the
time revealed a minor subdural bleed. No
neurological fallout. *Any trauma to the head is
significant and will have lifelong effects. We
see this during consultations as changes to the
physical body.*

Being *stretched* in life may not feel personally constructive at the time, but it often builds resilience in a person. Physically, mentally, emotionally, and spiritually, being *stretched* can induce changes that may strengthen you as a person, and you will be better off for it. And remember, *change is inevitable*[118].

Here is the truth. It will not be easy to gain flexibility. It

---

[118] This is about Concept seven in Chapter 5: *Muscles and joints need to be re-educated*. When we put a patient through a NRE protocol, it is only towards the last few weeks that we see the real change in flexibility (as an example). During the first three weeks, flexibility feels as if it gets worse. This is because the body resists change, until the brain is re-educated about what the *new normal* should feel like.

will most likely be painful at times and test your patience. And it almost certainly feels as if it gets worse before it gets better. The key to flexibility is that it is one of the body's superpowers of 'self -healing' and stretching is one of the mechanisms by which the body can pursue it.

After the New York City Marathon in 2019, I wanted to increase my flexibility. My flexibility was not bad, but I needed an *off-season* to really work on it. I needed some time off running, so after the marathon seemed like the perfect hiatus. I always explain to patients how functional gains (in things like flexibility, core strength, proprioception, or pain) often feel as if they get worse before they get better. I experienced that first-hand. Over a six-week period after the marathon I stretched all the muscles linked with hip mobility every day[119]. I warmed up properly and stretched. And I was in pain. My tendons were screaming at me. Groin pain, pelvic pain, you name it, I had it. I explain to patients how this amount of excessive stretching is damaging to the muscles and the tendons (which is a necessary evil for gaining flexibility). I felt it - believe me, I felt it. I was micro-tearing the structures every day, but here is the catch: provided you allow the muscles and tendons to repair, they will regenerate better than before.

Over the six-week period, new muscle tissue would have grown. Physiology 101. Again, I experienced all of that. My patience was tested when after a month of solid stretching, I was not more flexible at all. If anything, I was worse off. Until one day it all fell into place, and almost overnight I saw massive gains.

---

[119] I put myself through a NRE protocol for flexibility. What are the hip mobility muscles? To keep it simple, look at your leg; at the front of the leg you have your quads, outside is the glute and ITB, at the back of your leg are the hamstrings and inside are the adductors (groin). If you increase flexibility in these, you will have a better range of motion. In sport, this means more distance per stride (speed), and in patients this means less wear and tear (pain) in your spine.

And this catch is the basis for how muscles, ligaments and tendons heal. We introduce necessary trauma (treatment), and provided the body recovers properly, you will have gained a stronger structure than before. This is the same way that a healed broken leg is stronger than the original bone.

The body has a funny way of resisting change even though it is more than capable of doing so. We all resist change, some more than others, but we all know that change can be good. The body will resist until it recognizes the normal neuromusculoskeletal memory again.

What followed this flexibility phase of my life, was more pain. As I started running again, my lower back and pelvis started to ache. The only explanation I had for that was that now my pelvis was getting used to its new range of motion and its new flexibility. There was new inflammation and aggravation as the joint surfaces and ligaments that structurally hold my pelvis together underwent new mechanical forces. This went on for - you guessed it - six weeks. Six weeks of developing new neuromusculoskeletal memory but also the standard six weeks to repair strained structures with new tissue.

This speaks of the importance of Zone 2 exercise in this process.

We cannot all be as supple as leopards. If you want to be more flexible and adaptable, you must practice challenging your comfort zones. Of course, it is not an easy road, and it is certainly not pain free either. Flexibility takes time. It is like a leather belt, it eventually stretches, but it takes weeks and sometimes months of constantly applied small stretches.

There is an old saying that if you hang around the barber shop long enough, you will eventually get a haircut. If you stretch for a long enough time, you will eventually be more supple.

Let me explain the benefits of flexibility. You increase your functional range of motion while increasing blood flow to the effected joint and muscle. This decreases healing time and helps optimise the supercompensation phase of recovery (more about this later). Stretching after exercise allows muscles to cool down at length, which means they will warm up quicker when repeating the exercise[120].

Every Hour

I once saw an elderly patient whose main area for improvement was her flexibility. She specifically needed gluteal stretches and tennis ball ischaemic compressions; a fancy term for pushing the blood out of the muscles so that new blood can enter. Simply, tight muscles prevent blood flow.

My advice to her was to stretch every hour. I demonstrated to her how to do the stretch, my classic glute cues: *Sit on the edge of the chair. Cross your leg to put your ankle on your opposite knee. Most importantly, make yourself as tall as possible so that you keep a straight spine whilst leaning forward. You should feel a stretch. Now hold it until you feel the muscle stretch less and repeat it on the other side. Perform that simple routine every hour.*

A two-week follow-up consultation was set up. When she came in again, with all due respect, she looked like a wreck. She had bags under her eyes and appeared worse for wear. We normally expect good reports, so I was genuinely concerned when I asked what had happened. She went on to explain that she had been setting a cell phone alarm every hour to do the

---

[120] The muscle literally and figuratively does cool down. Also known as warming down. You are simply allowing the muscle to relax after strenuous exercise or excessive stretching. This allows blood to flow into it before you sit down and restrict blood flow to the muscle. Especially your leg muscles. This will help you recover quicker. In my experience: three to ten minutes is considered adequate. I will always try finish my run 500m from home and use the walk home as a cool down. This is where stretching after exercise is even more helpful: the muscle will relax at a stretched length as opposed to a shortened one.

stretches. By every hour I meant every hour OF THE DAY. She had been waking up every hour during the night to do her stretches. I was beyond impressed. I have never seen that kind of commitment before, but I explained to her that the hourly stretches related to waking hours only.

It was only during the Covid 19 lockdowns that I gained an understanding for office workers who said that they battle to perform their hourly stretches. *I mean, how hard can it be.* I did not buy their excuses, until I was that person. During the lockdown I was doing so much writing and editing, that I found myself sitting in the same position for two, sometimes three hours at a time. I had no excuse of stress or pressure from a boss; my motivator was more the pleasure of getting stuck into a task. So, I quickly learnt that you need to be two things: conscious and compliant. Conscious to set an alarm to remind you to get up, and compliant to stand up every hour and do suggested stretches. I would focus on the three stretches in the chapter *Good Posture and Slipping Discs.* (And I regularly joined the Hundreds Club.)

Another little trick is to drink plenty of water. Subsequently, you will need to make a few trips to the loo, and each time you do, do the stretches while you are up.

Flexibility is defined as the ability of a muscle to stretch and return to its normal length. It is not limited to long muscles, but to any muscle that can stretch and return to normal. The most important time to stretch would be after exercise[121].

---

[121] Remember earlier how nature reminds us of so many things. You would not put a racehorse away while it is wet, would you? You would walk it around for a while to allow the muscles to cool down at length. The same is true for humans. The most effective stretch is done when the muscle is warmed up, i.e. after a run.

In the posture chapter we spoke about how a short pectoral muscle will induce a tight trapezius muscle. The solution for that would be to stretch the pectorals before strengthening the trapezius. Similarly, thanks to our sitting culture, our deep hip flexors shorten, inducing muscle activation in our gluteal muscles and lower back extensors, merely to keep us upright when we are standing and walking. The only solution to that scenario is – yes, you guessed it – to stretch the hip flexors before strengthening the glutes and lower back.

These muscle imbalances develop a muscle memory, which, if you recall, is in fact a nerve memory in the motor cortex of our brains. Therefore, changing these imbalances takes time - time spent continually working on our flexibility, core, and posture, and continuing with these until they become the new nerve memories. I often explain to patients that we need to create a new normal so to say, so that when we do slouch or bend badly the body instantly feels that it is in an abnormal position. Eventually, this becomes almost subconscious.

A loss of flexibility may not seem like a big deal as we get older. It is normal to think that it is no longer necessary to do the kinds of athletic movements we did when we were younger. However, flexibility is the subtle trick that enables us to move safely and easily, and the way to stay flexible is to stretch. I do not think we always realize just how important stretching is for avoiding injury and disability. If you observe cats in nature, you will see that they are the only animals who stretch regularly. Consequently, their bodies last the longest (relative to other animals who do not naturally stretch and in relation to functional/ hunting ability before death).

Losing Flexibility

Flexibility naturally declines as the years go by because muscles become stiffer. The actin and myosin filaments that make up muscle tissue develop scar tissue, and they denature with age. If you do not keep stretching them, muscles will shorten. A shortened muscle does not contract as well as a muscle at its designed length. If you try utilizing a shortened muscle for activity, this will put you at risk for muscle tearing, strains, and joint sprains.

Warning signs that you are losing flexibility would be finding it difficult to put your shoes and socks on, or something as mundane as tucking in the back of your shirt.

Stretching Benefits

When you stretch a muscle, the muscle nears its full length[122]. If you hold that tension long enough, the muscle will be longer when it relaxes again. It is like stretching an elastic band - eventually the band will be slightly longer.

The important thing to remember here is that elastic bands will snap if stretched when they are cold. The only way to gain flexibility is very regular small stretches. A MoveMed stretching routine would include ten small stretches a day per desired muscle group. The more often you stretch your muscles, the more efficient and more flexible they become. As a result, you increase your range of motion; reduce your risk of muscle and joint injury; reduce joint and back pain; improve your balance, (thereby reducing your risk of falling); and improve your posture.

---

[122] That's what she said! You've already seen this a few times now. If you have ever watched the American version of *The Office*, you would have heard Michael Scott say that. If you have not watched it this is how it works. If something innocent could imply something inappropriately sexual, then you say *that's what she said*. And everyone sees the funny side. On an average day at the clinic, my work is full of these. *That feels so good*. Or. *Yes, that's the spot*. Or my favourite. *I wish the session were longer.*

The Power of Flexibility

Five-time Dance World Champion Chace Collett has experienced the benefits of stretching and flexibility throughout her career. From mobility, to posture, to muscle strength, to a positive mindset, she advocates stretching as an essential aspect of an exercise regime, whether you are an athlete or not. Unlike most of us, when Chace presented to the clinic as a patient, we found that in her case, being too flexible can cause its own set of injuries.

Chace is a special case. Many dancers are. I always joked with Chace that she had a *first world problem* in that too much flexibility became a risk factor for her injuries. In reality, this is not applicable to most patients. I have found that almost all patients lack flexibility somewhere in their bodies.

Here are a few examples, and these are a massive generalization. Hypothetically, if we could isolate flexibility as the only injury risk factor:

Laptop users often have short pectorals, leading to stiff necks. Office workers and desk users often have short hamstrings, leading to recurrent strains while running. Cyclists often have short hip flexors, leading to a stiff back. And runners have short glutes, leading to a multitude of injuries like shin splints, plantar fasciitis knee pain or low back pain.

The list goes on and on.

The important thing to understand is how flexibility plays a part in health. One of the goals of health is to restore normal movement - to move the way we were designed to move. To do this we need to stretch what is short, strengthen what is weak (previous chapter) and stabilize what is unstable (spoiler, the next chapter).

Point to ponder: Are you *stretching* yourself by trying to improve your flexibility?

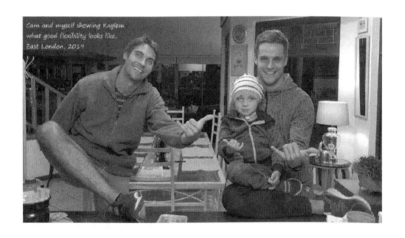

Cam and myself showing Kaylem what good flexibility looks like. East London, 2019

10 : Proprioception

Jon has not seen a chiropractor before. No
history of illnesses. *Rule out TIMID CAT
(Thyroid, inflammatory diseases, malignancy,
increased blood pressure, diabetes, cancer,
autoimmune diseases, trauma).*

To introduce the focus of this chapter, I would like
you to quickly stand up where you are. Now stand
on one leg and close your eyes. Your ankle is likely
to begin to shake or move from side to side. That, in a nutshell,
is called Proprioception. It is a nerve function whereby the
ligaments of the ankle tell your brain where you are in space.
It is an especially important function not to lose, and it is one
that we will benefit from if we can improve it.

Proprioception ties in closely with rehabilitation of sports
injuries. And sometimes you need to take a step back.

Wayde Van Niekerk is the reigning Olympic 400-metre
champion. His epochal moment came at the Olympic Games
in 2016 when he ran the fastest 400-meter race in history,
breaking a 17-year-old world record in the process. Defying

the odds and running from lane 8, he completed the single 400m lap in 43:03 seconds, beating the previous record set by Michael Johnson by 0.15 seconds. He also broke Johnson's 300-meter world record time.

This man, the fastest man in the world, injured his knee playing in a celebrity rugby match in Cape Town, South Africa, in October of 2017. He tore his anterior cruciate ligament and suffered medial and lateral tears of the meniscus. He underwent major surgery to repair his knee and his rehabilitation took months.

He documented parts of his rehabilitation process on social media, and I followed it closely. One of his recorded rehabilitation sessions showed him standing on one leg and learning to balance again. Proprioception 101. He needed to teach every structure and tissue how it is meant to fire, and this in turn reminded the part of his brain responsible for that movement what it was meant to be experiencing. Once he had done that, he could progress.

This is a profound reminder indeed of our body's mortality, seeing the fastest man in the world over 300 to 400 metres having to go back to basics. If even those that seem super-human need to do it, we need to just the same. The principle of proprioception is relative to any injury. Even if you have bruised a joint, you need to teach it again how it is meant to move. Often that will include some physical therapy to *get* the joint moving, and certainly some exercises to *keep* it moving.

As mentioned previously, I experienced this during my training for the New York Marathon. To train effectively, I had to take a step back and be patient.

Here is an example.

November 2017

Jessica Fletcher, a 73-year-old female presents to the clinic. Patient explains that she is familiar with solving murder cases, but this was a case she could not solve.

Jessica has mild low back pain. What grabs my attention is she described a fall she had FIVE YEARS prior to this consultation. She explains her visit to the hospital at the time and that their ONLY recommendation upon inspection of her X-rays was six weeks of bed rest. Patient recalls six weeks of excruciating bed rest, and eventually the pain settled. When she started moving again, she noticed that her left leg was not straight, and it was shorter[123].

We ruled out Legg-Calvé-Perthes disease (by default, as this hip problem is only seen in children between two and twelve years of age).

X-rays were justified and taken and reveal an obvious healed fracture of the neck of her femur (that is the kink in the thigh bone just before your hip ball and socket). We get hold of her X-rays from the original fall and we observe a clear telescoped fracture[124].

We are now dealing with a severe biomechanical problem and it would be too risky to operate to correct it. We pursued a NRE protocol. The patient lives a normal life now, with monthly maintenance treatments.

The good-to-knows:

ONE. Second opinions are always a good option.

TWO. You are never too old to start exercise.

---

[123] Alarm bells begin to ring if a patient describes this. Red flag. Similarly, a patient who describes that NOTHING had changed since applying the treatment protocol. I expect either to help with the patient's pain or to flare something up (which we now know is a good thing). When NOTHING changes, cancer is a possibility, and it is best to refer the patient - this has happened three times in my career so far.

[124] That is where the bone telescopes over itself because the internal integrity of the bone is non-existent. It is not the easiest fracture to see, as the bone is not blatantly displaced. Okay, I shall stop making excuses. That should have been picked up, especially by someone whose job it is to look for fractures in a fallen 80-something-year-old.

Running Shoes

I am often asked which running shoes are best for one's feet. Nike. Adidas. Brooks. Hoka. Sarcony? These are the most well-known brands it seems, and there are, of course, many more. My answer to this FAQ, however, is *whichever ones you think are the prettiest.* Or if I were getting paid to give an answer, it would be the brand who paid me. Jokes aside, the truth is that the brand of shoes you buy is irrelevant. I personally choose NIKE Pegasus running shoes because they have a simple swoosh, and I feel like Mo Farah when I wear them.

Before you ask the question of *which shoe is best*, you should answer for yourself: *have I done everything possible to strengthen my feet?* In particular, the integrity of the arch of your foot. In other words, *does your arch support itself?*

If yes, buy the pretty shoes or the ones that make you feel like Hercules. If no, get to work on yourself before you part with your money and place high expectations on a pair of shoes. If your feet are strong, then completely worn-out shoes are better for you than new expensive arch-supported shoes.

In essence, if the stability and arches of your feet are strong (and the terrain you were training on was not damaging), running barefoot would be best for your feet, and shoes merely an aesthetic accessory. Studies have been conducted on brain activity when we walk barefoot as opposed to when we walk wearing shoes. It is staggering to see how the brain scan lights up like a Christmas tree when we are barefoot. We are starving our brains of sensory input just by wearing shoes for prolonged time.

So, the question now is: *how do you strengthen your feet?* Answer: Proprioception.

I have performed countless health experiments on myself. One of them is using the same pair of Nike's Pegasus 33 for more than three years and hundreds of running kilometres. I still have the shoes, and if you could see them, the best word to describe them would be *grotty*. There is barely any tread on them, and zero cushion arch support. This particular health experiment was to test if a lack of cushioning related to injuries. Touch wood, they did not.

If shoe arch support was as essential as the marketing said it was, I should have had numerous injuries. My only hypothesis from this health experiment is that if we strengthen the ligament integrity of our feet (proprioception), our shoe cushioning or arch support is irrelevant.

Falls

An underrated benefit of proprioception is the decreased risk of falls. It is particularly valuable among elderly patients who have an increased risk of fracture when falling. In terms of fitness, the benefit is decreased risk of sports injuries. Additionally, and this applies to all of us, there is the benefit of stronger joints, meaning that there is less chance of developing arthritis - or at least the effects of arthritis are minimised.

Receptors, called proprioceptors are found in the skin, joints, ligaments, tendons, and muscles. The receptors receive signals indicating the position, orientation, and movement of the body, and this information is directed to the brain. The brain then uses this information to create a constantly changing map of your position, called *Position Sense*.

Joints are managed by a specific section in the brain. When a joint has stopped moving, there is no signal to the brain for that specific joint. The part of the brain responsible for that joint switches off. We witness that in treatment. When a joint that has not been active for a while starts moving, it takes time to keep itself moving.

A practical example of this is the way a patient responds to a six-week NRE protocol. The patient comes in for regular treatment and for the first few weeks the joints are as restricted (not moving) as their first assessment. This is because there was an absent neuromusculoskeletal memory for months to years, and the brain forgot what that stimulation felt like. Towards the end of a six-week NRE protocol, we usually see that patients begin to *hold* their adjustments. During any treatment protocol, we give exercises and stretches, which is primarily to help maintain the movement we have restored during treatment. Eventually the brain identifies this as normal again, and we start seeing the patient drastically less once this has happened. Proprioception (coupled with Zone 2 training as we saw earlier) is the most effective ways of re-educating joints to function the way they are meant to function once normal movement has been restored.

We all naturally need to improve our balance and our proprioception, particularly when we consider the detrimental effect of shoes on our proprioception. When we sprain our ankles, it is important to restore ankle function as soon as possible after the injury. An injured ligament will lose its proprioceptive function as a protective mechanism to force you to limp and therefore take pressure off the injury. Re-educating the ankle to support itself is a key goal in the rehabilitation. Chronic ankle instability, caused by inadequate rehabilitation and healing after a sprain, can result in increasingly injurious sprains, arthritis, or tendon problems.

One form of proprioceptive exercise is basic balance training which has been shown to prevent lower limb ligament re-injury and reduce the risk of ligament problems in athletes. If it works for athletes, imagine what it does for the rest of us.

It may be easier than you think to add proprioceptive balance training into your daily routine. Try some of the following activities:

Stand on one leg whenever you are waiting in line at the post office, bank, food store or even while brushing your teeth.

Stand on a piece of foam or folded towel during a break at work or whenever you are on the phone.

Practice catching a tennis ball while standing on one leg. (You can throw it against the wall.)

Practice sitting down and getting up from a chair without using your hands.

Practice walking heel to toe, placing the heel of one foot just in front of the toes of the opposite foot each time you take a step.

Visit the MoveMed YouTube channel and follow the proprioception video.

Sport

One aspect of proprioception is purely feet strengthening. The reason for this being that many of us have weakening feet because we grew up wearing shoes. Remember, *if you do not use it, you lose it*. If you consistently have arch support supporting your feet, you will not need your own body's support. Another aspect of improving one's proprioception is that when an injury happens, it could be less severe even if your proprioception is only almost adequate.

Here is an example.

I mentioned earlier that I competed in Lifesaving. My best event was the two kilometre beach run[125]. It was always a dream of mine to win an individual national title. I am sure any sportsperson has the same dream. The national science Olympiad title I won did not count as I competed as part of a team of three. They say there is no "I" in *team*. Well, there is an "I" in *win*. I had not won an individual title yet.

---

[125] There are only six lifesaving events. Three water and three land events. Of the three land events, I only participated in the 100m sprint - thanks for those genes' mom, and the two kilometre beach run - thanks for those genes' dad. It was always expected of us to participate in all the events. For the whole *vibe*. I only took part in my two land events, and hence got the name *Bolt* at the East London Surf Lifesaving Club.

The lead up to the 2017 nationals was epic. The previous year, at the 2016 nationals, I had badly strained my hamstring in the 100m beach sprints event where I somehow managed a silver medal. I therefore could not participate in the 2016 two kilometre beach run, my main event, which was two days later, on the final day of competition. I had a bone to pick with 2017 and therefore I was focused. I was eating clean and training hard. This was another health experiment for me: I was properly focussing on the MoveMed rehabilitation concepts. And it worked. I was in the best shape of my life, physically, mentally, and spiritually.

A good indicator is when running feels like gliding as opposed to feeling like dragging your body through the mud. The 2017 nationals were held in Camps Bay, Cape Town. It is an idyllic beach at the base of Table Mountain - there could not have been a better setting to potentially attain my goal.

A two kilometre beach race is interesting to say the least. The conditions can be so variable. You can have hard sand, which essentially makes it a track race. You can have soft sand, which is not pretty to watch, it looks like pain in slow motion. Or you can have a mixture of hard and soft sand sections depending on the high and low tides.

But this is where the story gets exciting. Two weeks before the race I decided to go for a trail run with Don (my cousin who you will become more acquainted with in the chapter *Eat Clean*). Running down a sweeping sharp left turn, my right ankle got caught in a tree root. My entire momentum continued downwards, and my body ripped over my right ankle. I heard a loud pop in the ankle before slamming into the ground on my right shoulder. I tumbled down the hairpin corner. I immediately knew something was wrong. The involuntary yelp I made, caused Don to stop and come find me. (Don is normally in front.)

Whenever I fall, the first thing I check is my collar bone. I felt around my chest to make sure nothing was sticking through my skin. I performed a few shoulder shrugs to make sure I had no broken clavicle. Next, I assessed my ankle. There was no blood or bone sticking out. I did a few ankle circles, and it felt fine. The most important test, *can I bear weight* (stand on it)? I could. Relief!

I knew I had damaged my ligaments, which meant I could walk home. Don and I were four kilometres from his house. I tied my laces as tightly as possible and started my careful walk home. By the time we reached Don's house the ankle was twice its normal size. I applied some ice immediately and headed home. By that stage, my ankle was black and blue.

Grading ligament injuries is easy. Grade 1 is an ankle sprain, clear by moderate swelling. Typically, two weeks for recovery and treatment is needed to get it back to normal. A black and blue ankle (with ankle strength) indicates a Grade 2 tear. This is what I had, and it typically requires six weeks for recovery and treatment to return to normal functioning. Grade 3 ligament injuries cause black and blue bruising alongside a loss of ankle strength (in other words your ligament has completely torn off the bone, hence the lack of strength), and this would probably require surgery to fix.

With a Grade 2 tear I should have been out of sport for six weeks and would have kissed my national title hopes goodbye. Instead of the expected outcome of six weeks of recovery, I was on the elliptical trainer (sky runner) one week later. The following week I won my first National Championship title.

The good-to-knows:

ONE. There may have been some miracle healing that took place. I cannot prove that.

TWO. If my ankles were not strong from actively focusing on proprioception exercises, I would have been out of action for six weeks. Or worse, I could have torn the ligament completely which would have resulted in surgery.

THREE. Prevention (when possible) is better than cure.

FOUR. Do not be an idiot like me and go for a technical trail run two weeks before any competition.

Not Just for Athletes

As mentioned earlier, balance training helps reduce the risk of falls in older adults with balance problems, and for anyone with low bone mass. It also improves postural stability after a stroke.

As is to be expected, our balance tends to get worse with time, especially if we are not active. Inactivity causes neural connections to be lost if they are not used. So, whether you want to recover from an ankle sprain or maintain your long-term health, proprioception exercises should be on your 'To-Do' list.

The great thing about proprioception training is that you do not need a lot of equipment and training to perform the basics. It all starts with good posture, which you can practice almost anytime, anywhere.

The basic idea is to start stabilizing your body under increasingly difficult circumstances or on uneven surfaces. For example, balance on one leg - first on a flat hard floor, then on a soft surface like foam or a folded up towel, progressing to a bosu ball or wobble board , and eventually on to a bosu ball or wobble board while catching a ball or receiving a push to your shoulder from different angles[126].

---

[126] A wobble board is normally a flat circular piece of wood with a rounded object attached to the center of it. If you place the board on the ground with the rounded object touching the floor, the board will lean to one side. By standing on the board, you attempt to balance in such a way as to not let the board touch the floor. It looks like a mixture of surfing and snowboarding. A bosu ball is half of an inflatable gym ball, attached to a hard-circular base. The same principle as above applies while the hard surface is facing upwards. The bosu ball can also be placed hard surface down, and you can attempt to balance on the soft inflatable half ball. These exercises are great to strengthen your balance, and more specifically your proprioception.

Keep it Simple

I often sound like a broken recorder, always stressing flexibility, core activations and Proprioception to my patients. But the truth is that these three are the fundamentals of any movement. Imagine you had hip replacement. You now have brand new hip joint that needs to learn how to move. This is the rawest form of rehabilitation. Now go and imagine that you have not had a joint replacement, yet you applied the same rehabilitation protocol. The joint will only move better, further, stronger and more efficiently. This is when we start to delve into performance enhancement - the free and legal kind, not the kind Lance made a few headlines for.

Point to ponder: Prevention (whenever possible) is better than cure.

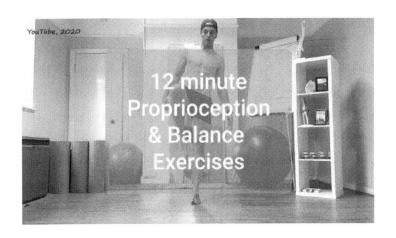

YouTube, 2020

12 minute
Proprioception
& Balance
Exercises

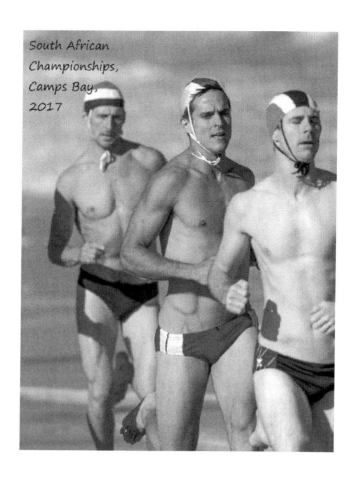

South African
Championships,
Camps Bay,
2017

11 : Recovery, Sleep and Off-seasons

Jon explains a family history of disc injuries.
His father had two lumbar spine fusions.
Mother suffers with migraines and clinically
diagnosed depression. *Does not mean he will
suffer these. Control what you can control.*

How we recover has an impact on our health and wellbeing in every way imaginable. If I could say that one area of health is essential for survival, it would be recovery. It may sound obvious, but without proper recovery we would die from a simple bruised muscle. I am convinced that recovery us one of the great secrets to a healthy life; and reaching this epiphany came during a stage of my learning I call: The Great Realisation.

I have become somewhat single-minded about the concept of recovery, and those close to me will confirm that I regularly check and speak about my resting heart rate and why I feel I should not stay out late too often. I know the effect it will have on my body, and I do not think it is because I am growing old - 31 is, after all, young (right?).

Life is a balance between recovery and movement. Essentially, by recovery, I mean 'eat, sleep, *move,* repeat[127]' - eat clean, sleep enough and exercise. Recovery is the most unappreciated tool that we all have and very few people realise its significance. It is a simple equation, recovery is directly proportional to fitness, fitness is directly proportional to burnout prevention, and burnout prevention is directly proportional to injury risk.

Let me paint you a picture, using a case study.

January 2018

Phoebe Buffay, a 33-year-old female, presented to the clinic. Phoebe has many friends who are giving her mixed advice. She is a way above average runner who was training for a marathon in six weeks' time.

Phoebe lives out of town and therefore I was able to see her only every fortnight. Patient injured her gastrocnemius, one of her calf muscles, while running. Her injury was a Grade 1 strain. We were faced with a super tight band of calf tissue that needed to heal quickly.

This is how we grade muscle strains (and it is almost identical to how we grade ligament strains as we saw in the previous chapter): Grade 1 strain means that the muscle fibres came close to tearing but the body spasmed to prevent that happening. A Grade 2 strain has torn muscle fibres. Grade 3 is complete rupture of the muscle, that you can hear when it

---

[127] "Eat, Sleep, Rave, Repeat" is a song by Fatboy Slim, Riva Starr and Beardyman. It features vocals from Beardyman who improvised all the lyrics and vocals in one take.

happens. When a rugby player tears a hamstring during a game, it often sounds like a pop, a loud crack. It is as though a sniper has shot the player because he reacts as though he has been shot in the leg.

Duchenne muscular dystrophy was ruled out and I explained that eccentric muscle loading was what injured the muscle. For two weeks Phoebe would need to avoid that[128].

The advice given to Phoebe was that she undertakes a MoveMed rehabilitation and cross training programme for two weeks. Stretching, core and cross training would be safe for the niggle, and I explained that she would not lose any fitness as she could still do cardiovascular intervals. Running however, would need to be avoided for two weeks.

An example of cross training is the sky runner machine that is offered at most indoor and outdoor gyms. It is a highly underrated piece of fitness equipment I trained solely on the sky runner for an off-road marathon while I was nursing a niggle. Not only does one gain fitness on the sky runner, but all the same running muscles are activated in a slightly different way. It is like having an off-season without losing aerobic fitness, which is invaluable for a sportsperson.

I stressed numerous times to Phoebe the imperative that she avoid running for two weeks. I saw Phoebe two weeks later, and she had strained the calf yet again - running of course. It was a Grade 1 strain again and I gave the same speech. I saw Phoebe another two weeks later, which was now two weeks before her marathon, but this time she had completely torn her calf muscle, a Grade 2 strain, while running of course. The prognosis now was not good. The immense bruising extending

---

[128] Eccentric muscle load is when the muscle is contracting against force, and the force is larger than the contraction. The muscle is lengthening against the load. During running, this happens as the heel lands on the ground. Picture it - the calf lengthens against force to try and slow our body weight down. The calf then helps to control our movement before momentum brings our centre of gravity over the foot again and then to propel us forward. Running biomechanical assessments can become very intense.

into her ankle meant that she would definitely not be able to run her marathon. She dealt with the disappointment and we eventually became friends again.

The good-to-knows:

ONE. Create a healing environment for the injury to heal.

TWO. Cross training is wonderfully beneficial - it is like a mini off-season, where you gain or maintain fitness without causing new injuries.

THREE. Do not underestimate real recovery.

In sport, you can only train as hard as your recovery allows. In healthcare, it is the same. You will not heal or recover if the body is stressed and if there is not an environment for healing to take place.

Fitness is a rather simple concept, one that I have tried and tested myself over the last few years. Interestingly, I have found that the word 'fitness' can be used interchangeably with the word 'health'. Recovery, or how much you recover, determines the rate and efficiency at which the body can heal and adapt to previous stressors or injuries.

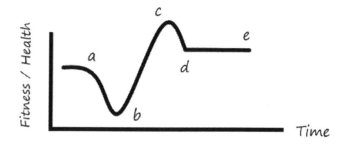

Fitness Over Time

Let me explain the graphic above in terms of your fitness. The dark line is your instantaneous fitness level. If you exercise (a), your fitness will immediately drop the same day directly after the exercise (b). An example of this is if you try running ten kilometres in the afternoon after running ten kilometres that morning. Your body will be fatigued, which represented in the first dip of the graph. Over the next two days your body will recover and gain a fitness far greater than you had before. The gain in fitness is called supercompensation (c) and is one of the body's natural processes to deal with stress, which is shown as the bump in the graph after the dip. After this, your body will settle at a new fitness level (d) that is directly proportional to how much recovery you have had. In the graph above, this is higher/ better (e) than the starting fitness (a). Net fitness gain is achieved only with adequate recovery.

Health Over Time

Now let me explain the graph above in terms of health. The dark line is your instantaneous health or immune system level (a). If you have a stress, overuse injury or viral infection, for example, your health will deteriorate, as shown as the dip in the graph (b). Over the next few days, your body will recover and regain a health greater than you had before (supercompensation), as shown by the bump (c). Your body will then settle at a new health level (d) that is directly proportional to how much recovery you have had. In this theoretical graph above, the new health is greater than before (e). I have found this to be true throughout my own health journey, one example of this being my recovery from hepatitis.

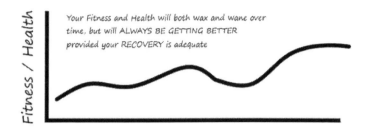

The graph above is what our lives *should* look like. All the dips in the graph are days when the body has not recovered from the previous day's exercise or stress. You can identify this by using your resting heart rate[129]. The rises in the graph indicate the body compensating or adapting to the previous day's exercise or stress. The rises mean that your body is in a healing environment and this is our goal. Overall, the projection of your health and fitness is upwards - always improving[130].

---

[129] The next chapter speaks about how to do this effectively. It is a simple skill to master and a skill that could change the flight path of your health journey for the better.

[130] This view of health in a linear way is to illustrate how our bodies recover and get healthier, stronger, etc. Keep it simple. The *KISS principle* from earlier. Black or white. You are either always improving (healing) or you are slowly getting worse. There is of course also a top plateau of health that one reaches, and a bottom plateau (called death). Until such plateaus, we all tend to yo-yo up and down throughout our lives. That said, the healthiest people can drop dead from a heart attack that may not be health related at all, but rather a neurological mishap which we have no control over. Therefore, I always say control what you can control. And if you do, as these graphs show, your health trajectory tends to be upwards or downwards over a long period of time.

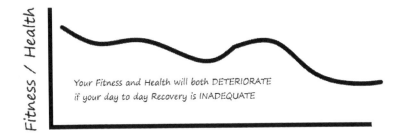

Your Fitness and Health will both DETERIORATE
if your day to day Recovery is INADEQUATE

The above graph is what our lives should hopefully never look like. The dips in the graph are days when the body has NOT recovered from the previous day's exercise or stress. Due to inadequate recovery the body's compensation and adaption are not enough. In real life this looks like the following:

May 2018

Thomas Shelby, a 35-year-old male presents to the clinic. A local politician and avid runner, he has been attending the clinic for five years.

Over this time, Thomas has recorded, on average, six to eight bouts of flu per year. In this same period, he has recorded an average of six episodes of low back pain and three episodes of medial knee pain that warranted treatment, per year.

We ruled out pot (the drug), POTS (postural orthostatic tachycardia syndrome), and the other Potts which is Tuberculosis of the spine.

We performed a retrospective informal assessment of his training habits over the last five years as this was his primary risk factor. He records on average, one "easy" training session per week out of six sessions. He did not use a heart rate monitor or any specific training program. We discuss this and agree that his "easy" session would have been a Zone 2 effort.

Thomas agrees to a more structured training style and "non-painful treatments"[131]. He invests in a heart rate monitor and we spend three months adjusting his training program to fit his lifestyle. A year later, I have seen him for monthly check-ups. In a year, he has experienced only one episode of low back pain and two episodes of knee pain.

The good-to-knows:

ONE. Around 80% of his training sessions were always Zone 3 and higher - he was getting negligible levels of recovery, if any. He had a stressful job, and his training habits were only adding stress to his body.

TWO. Over 80% of his training should have been in Zone 2.

THREE. One cannot change a five-year habit overnight; one changes it with baby steps. The next step is for Thomas to start some proprioception training. Rome was not built in a day, neither is a healing environment.

I know what you are thinking, cute story, but how do we recover?

There are many ways to recover *better*. First and foremost, a recovery-focused lifestyle can be achieved best by working alongside a Health Coach. The guidance of a Health Coach not only keeps you accountable but facilitates physical treatment, *Neural Re-Education*, and risk identification. I will elaborate on this in the chapters that follow.

---

[131] This means he will come in for 'maintenance' treatments. Many patients use the word "maintenance" and when they do, I do not correct them. Although I prefer the word "check-ups" as treatment sometimes has a negative connotation to it. Essentially, we treat "before the injuries happen". This is where I want every patient to be. And this is not a sales pitch. I undergo treatment once a month. I believe everyone should. And every month I am as *locked up* as the previous month. *Locked up* referring to areas of the body that stop moving owing to our 21st century lifestyles. Therefore, I am so passionate about this because I am living proof of this system. *Move how you were designed to move.*

Secondly, one of the most effective forms of recovery at home is Zone 2 exercise. Alongside this, it is important to fuel your body with the ingredients to build and repair cells in the form of good clean eating. Generous water intake and a healthy diet play a pivotal role in recovery. Then there is something we take for granted - getting enough sleep.

Sleep

Making sufficient sleep a priority can not only add years to your life, but it means that you also have a shorter workday. I reckon that might be a strong motivation for some people, so let us roll with it.

The most basic form of recovery is sleep. Your body releases growth hormone when you sleep; when you sleep, you heal. Reduced sleep has been linked to increased injury rates during athletic competitions. A University of California study concluded that injury rates in youth athletes increased during games that followed a night of fewer than six hours sleep. Another study looking at injury rates in high school athletes found that sleep hours were the strongest predictor of injuries, even more so than hours of practice[132].

What if I told you that I had a treatment that would reduce the internal body chemistry associated with stress; that would naturally increase human growth hormone; that would enhance recovery rate; and that would improve performance? The treatment is sleep - it does all those things.

For some reason, it has become popular for many people to try and get by on less sleep. I hear it all the time. *"I need only four hours sleep a night"*. Such little sleep is likely to add up

---

[132] The other day my 13-year-old cousin finished his exams. All he wanted to do to celebrate this feat was to stay up for 24 hours. I remember being that age and doing the same thing. Sometimes now, in celebration of something, I get an early night. What a treat.

to a real health problem. Many of us might already know that poor sleep is linked to diseases like heart attacks, strokes, and diabetes. What is equally serious is that poor sleep can cause depressive symptoms, make us act impulsively and be more sensitive to our own pain. It is not so surprising that we have difficulty relating to others and being the best version of ourselves when we are short of sleep.

Scientists are now starting to understand how not only the quantity, but also the quality of sleep impacts on our health and well-being. I have found that exercise and eating clean drastically improve the quality of my sleep. Mindfulness, and thinking outside of one's self has also proven to benefit my sleep, perhaps giving love simply opens your mind to sleeping soundly. It does not hurt to try.

Bedrest and sleep are quite different. Sleep will help you recover faster. When it comes to mechanical injuries, bedrest is a myth. You need to keep the body moving. Even patients in severe pain, would benefit from moving as soon as possible. And remember, walking is moving. Therefore, even during times that you have been advised bedrest, getting up every hour and walking around could also be beneficial.

As you get older, you need to recover more. I am sure we have all experienced this. Think back to when you were in your early twenties and you could party until the early hours of the morning. And some of us would do that a few nights in a row. Fast forward a few years , and one late night demands two good nights' rest to catch up.

Off-seasons

Another form of recovery is having an off-season. Professional athletes do it, but we amateurs often forget to structure it into our training or our lives. Not only athletes need off-seasons, everyone does. The off-season must be the most imperative season of an athlete's career.

At the clinic, I try to incorporate an off-season mentality into my patients' regimens of treatment. We all need to structure time into our year to have an off-season. Often, I would try to get patients to focus on a certain area of weakness for a few weeks at a time (flexibility, core, proprioception etc.). At the same time I would explain to them that this now makes them 'professional athletes', and this always helps with the motivation to get started.

An example of poor planning is running clubs which literally run all year around. There is often no clear off-season like professional athletes have[133]. All you need is two to six weeks of a different stimulus to the body to allow recovery to happen. It is the overload principle – the body will adapt to any new stimulus. Off-seasons are the only time to work on weaknesses you may have. An example would be flexibility. It is exceedingly difficult to gain flexibility as a runner during a running season, as the increased muscle aggravation while stretching means you are highly likely to tear a muscle.

Interestingly, I am writing this chapter amid a global pandemic, where I am witnessing, via social media, a huge number of people having a forced off-season. It seems that most people are being productive and doing something for their health, and their bodies are loving the new stimulation.

Even just a change in environment does wonders for your body. It allows certain aspects of your life to recover while you introduce an overload of new stimuli.

March 2020

Rachel Green, a 30-year-old female presents to the clinic.

---

[133] In the running clubs' defence, they cannot accommodate individual schedules. The onus should be on the individual. Running all year round means that runners should take their own off-seasons throughout the year based on their own fitness regimes.

Rachel has been attending the clinic for a year now. She has shown slow but progressive improvements. She is a London trader at a well-known firm, and she works a twelve-hour day on a stressful trading floor.

Rachel was coming for her monthly session. She explains that she has been working from home for three weeks (Covid 19 lockdown).

She explains that the three weeks in 'lockdown'[134] were "the best thing that could have ever happened to her". We rule out an acute psychotic episode and see that she is not imagining these things.

She feels less stressed. Her lingering cough has cleared up. She has more energy. Her sex life with her husband has improved. She ate healthier because she could prepare meals at home as opposed to eating office food for most meals. She lost weight.

The good-to-knows:

ONE. Her sudden improvement spike was from a forced period of different stimulation, and some extra movement. Less commute stress and zero commute time means she was able to do 30 minutes of exercise every day and sleep in an extra hour, all during the time she saved on commuting alone. Before the lockdown, she literally did not have the time. After three weeks of just those two changes (more sleep and some exercise coupled with less commute), she is, she says, a "new person".

---

[134] The Covid-19 lockdowns happened in most countries in the year 2020. It was a weird year to say the least. Companies had to restructure and people who could, were working from home for the foreseeable future. It was a weird year in the sense that some people flourished with this shock to the routine, and some went off the rails. Whether you like it or not, your perception of 'normal' life was rocked. As with this case in point, office workers would now work from home. This meant saving money and time on commuting. This meant being forced to prepare food for yourself as opposed to canteen or café meals. This meant more time for potential exercise and potential good healthy food habits. *Potential* is the key word there, as many people did not capitalise on this.

TWO. You do not need a lockdown to make some lifestyle changes, start by finding just ten minutes per day.

Prioritize Recovery

I think it is important that I practice what I preach. I will often put myself through a complete off-season. This will consist of two or three weeks of no running, with only core proprioception and flexibility training. When I originally wrote this chapter, I had just come back from the New York City marathon, and for the three weeks that followed I worked exclusively on core, proprioception and flexibility. I allowed my joints to heal after the race. You can feel when your body has been put through a significant trauma (which any marathon runner will tell you). Your body aches. Your joints are painful for days. You may be thinking: *How can that be good for you?*

Well the great realisation for me is this: *RUNNING IS NOT BAD FOR YOU.* But the imperative addition that must be attached to that statement is *PROVIDED YOUR RECOVERY IS ADEQUATE.* (In other words, *PROVIDED MOST OF YOUR RUNNING IS IN ZONE 2.*)

The same is true for illness, injuries, and traumas - traumas such as physical traumas (car accidents and sports injuries), chemical traumas (years of poor diet) or emotional ones (psychological hurt of any kind). All these together are not bad for you, *PROVIDED YOUR RECOVERY IS ADEQUATE.* You will be stronger for them, better, faster, more secure, and more confident subsequently, provided you spend the time healing.

And the key to this is patience. You can have it all, but you cannot have it all at once. (Despite what Freddie Mercury sang in one of the more famous Queen songs.) This is the basis for healing, and this is the basis for fitness - prioritize recovery. And together these are the foundations of health.

Point to ponder: Do you need to prioritise recovery a bit more in your life?

12 : Listen to Your Heart

We ruled out that Jon is not one of the Jumping Frenchmen of Maine. *I cannot even make these names up. This is an actual and extremely rare disorder characterized by extreme, involuntary and rapid startling reactions.*

The human heart is a piece of great ambiguity. Although it has no eyes, it can see your health's future. It has no mouth, yet it can tell you about the quality of your recovery. It has no brain, although the brain controls it, and it is the craftiest organ in the human body. This is a chapter on heart rate and this stage of learning is called: Being an idiot.

Have you ever thought just how intricately linked your health and your fitness are? Or what the single best thing is that you can do for your health? If you have, I have hopefully answered these questions in the previous chapter. Ultimately, the single answer to both questions, is *recovery*.

Over the years, I have studied textbooks, cut cadavers, touched bodies, and clinically treated and worked with patients to understand the human body. What we have is a wonderfully designed living biological system, that is designed to heal itself. If you take away the right stressors, *voila,* there is healing. Add more stressors to the system and you have injury, illness, or pain. With enough patience, passion, perseverance, a few sacrifices, and the correct mind set, you can achieve long term health and fitness, or at the very least, add healthy years to your life.

Healing will come to you from the unlikeliest of sources. By *unlikely* I mean that healing is simple, and we often overcomplicate things. Google will offer literally millions of opinions to help healing take place. Remember the *KISS* principle from Chapter Five? Remove excess inflammation and stress from your body and healing has a better chance of occurring. By tracking your resting heart rate, you can engage in a precise form of communication with your body and listen when it indicates its need for you to *take it easy*[135].

Over the last four years I have learnt how to read my resting heart rate. Originally, I took my pulse first thing in the morning, holding my two fingers against my neck, counting the beats for fifteen seconds, and then multiplying by four. However, I found that this was fairly inaccurate as I tended to always round up or round down. I therefore resolved to invest in a Garmin Fenix 5s sports watch with a wrist heart rate detector. Sleeping with it on allows you to obtain the most accurate resting heart rate over a night's sleep.

Your average resting heart rate will tell you a detailed story about what your body is doing in terms of recovery and

---

[135] My mother always told me to wear my heart on my sleeve. That became quite literal when I purchased a heart rate monitor. I have not found a more practical way to test personal recovery than a true base resting heart rate.

vulnerability to illness.

For example, if you observe a sudden spike in your resting heart rate (let us say your normal resting HR is 60 and all of a sudden it is 68), it tells you that your body has not recovered properly from the previous day. If you have not recovered completely from the previous day's stress (physical, mental, chemical etc.), you will then be at risk of falling ill or suffering an overuse injury if you train hard[136].

Similarly, if you wake up and your resting heart rate is lower than normal, it is fair to assume that your body has fully recovered, and you can theoretically train hard that day or that your general risk of illness is low.

I have found that because of monitoring my resting heart rate and guiding my exercise accordingly, I do not catch colds or fall ill anymore, or very rarely so. If my resting heart rate has risen, that day will be a full rest day or a stretch day, with lots of water, clean eating, and an early night of sleep.

This leads me on to the next topic, about which I am extremely passionate.

Zone 2

To explain the crux of Zone 2 (again) and why it is so important, let me use the following example. If I wake up and

---

[136] A quick check in. When we speak about stress, there are many kinds of stress. Physical stress: speaks for itself and this is what we do *to* our bodies, and includes any physical irritation to the nervous system - things like bad posture that overload muscles, overuse from too much exercise and not enough recovery, too many Red Zone efforts, not enough Zone 2 exercise, etc. It can also include what we *do not do to* our bodies (core exercise, flexibility, proprioception etc.). Chemical stress: this is what we put *into* our bodies, and there is an entire chapter dedicated to this later. Emotional stress: this refers to the subconscious stress *inside* our minds that we all have, from work, family, and relational internal conflicts, that ultimately leads to a prolonged (almost constant) fight or flight stress reaction, all thanks to the hormone cortisol.

my heart rate has risen by more than five beats per minute, I will have an easy Zone 2 training day, stretching alone or a rest day that day. If my training program for that day included a high intensity run or cycle, I will still do the run or cycle, except that it would be done in Zone 2.

In other words, if my resting heart rate in the morning is more than normal (compared to my personal average resting heart rate), I will prioritize recovery that day. An elevated or raised resting heart rate tells you that your body has not recovered (from something).

I first learnt about zones of exercise in the sports world from Dr Stephen Seiler, an American exercise physiologist. He described three training zones: Green, Orange and Red. Based on these findings, many other exercise platforms have described five zone models (Zone 1 to Zone 5), but it all boils down to these three broad zones - the Green Zone (Zone 1 and Zone 2); the Orange Zone (or Zone 3); and the Red Zone (Zones 4 and 5).

There are so many different coaching styles and wellness programs pertaining to fitness and health, where do you start? You pick one. Or you keep it simple.

Two Zone System

The MoveMed approach to exercise and wellness simply has two zones: Zone 2 and the Red Zone. The Two Zone System is that which I followed for my New York City 'fun-run' detailed in the second chapter and the one I recommend to my patients and athletes. The beauty of the Two Zone System is that it is a health formula that can be applied to any existing program or lifestyle. Also, it is simple. And we like to keep things simple.

Recover when you need to recover. Push hard when you need to push hard.

Everything that is not done in Zone 2 is afflictive to the

body; breaking parts of it down. The crux of the health philosophy I recommend is - breaking part of the body down (for example, the muscles during exercise or the joints' ligaments during chiropractic adjustments) is not detrimental, provided your recovery is adequate. That last part is most essential. Adequate recovery is key to repair any damage to muscles, tendons, or ligaments. Adequate recovery tilts the healing seesaw (Concept Two: *Create a healing environment* in Chapter 5) in our favour.

If you perform running sprints and Red Zone efforts, muscles and tendons in your body break down.

If I adjust a patient's neck or back, the ligaments and capsules of the joint break down.

If you do not *eat clean*, the chemical stressors from unhealthy foods break the body down internally (by adding excess inflammation).

If you have too much work-related stress in your life (most of us do), emotional stressors and cortisol break the body down.

All these examples increase inflammation in your body. Inflammation causes pain, and too much inflammation prevents healing, which is why Zone 2 is so important. That is why we should perform Zone 2 intensity for above 80% of our exercise regimes, because Zone 2 promotes recovery and recovery promote healing.

Years of data gathered by Dr Seiler show that most professional athletes are spending 80% to 90% of their training in Zone 2. Why do professionals do it, yet we do not? This was the question that baffled me, and one that prompted me to investigate this method in depth. A few years later I experienced, the importance of Zone 2 for sport.

During training with Olympians Oscar Pistorius and Martin Rooney in 2013, I experienced the importance of Zone 2 training for sport. We performed five 300-meter running sprints at around 40 seconds each. Out of a 90-minute session, we discharged three minutes of Red Zone effort; that is less than 5% of the session. Mostly, the session consisted of specific athletics drills aimed at warming up certain muscle groups, *teaching* the muscles certain firing patterns, exercise band work to further reiterate the muscle firing patterns and cooling down the entire body. I did not realise at the time, but we were developing a base - a neuromusculoskeletal base. An example of the essence of Neural Re-Education.

Fast forward a few more years. I thought I knew it all, and therefore, learnt that pride is the burden of a foolish person. Earlier in the book, I introduced you to my coach at the time, Clinton, and mentioned his involvement in my training for the New York Marathon. When we met, I was the classic Zone 3 athlete; every session was run at a fast-ish pace, somewhere between easy and all out. I would chase down anyone I saw running casually ahead of me or run with my brother which always ended up running too quickly[137]. Sure, you lose weight and stay lean running moderately hard every day. You will *get fit,* but you will not increase your speed by much, and, from my experience, you will pick up niggles - regular aches and pains, shin splints, knee pain, and back pain.

Clint told me very directly that I was an idiot and taught me practically about avoiding too much time spent exercising *just* outside of Zone 2. Clint taught me simply not to train *just* outside of Zone 2, rather make a non-Zone 2 session count by going hard or going home[138]. The entire next chapter is

---

[137] When I lived near my brother, Kaylem and I would run together most days. He would always say *"Let's do the big loop!"*. I would always say *"Let's do the small loop!"*. I would always be saying *"Slow down"*. He would always reply with a *"You suck"*. We would compromise with a medium paced, big loop, run.

[138] Remember, at MoveMed we like to keep things simple. Two zone system. You are either helping yourself heal or you are helping yourself hurt. When we say, *"just outside of Zone 2"*, that is the same as Zone 3 or the Orange Zone. This is the most pointless intensity to train at because you are getting all the negative aspects of *mildly* exerting your body (adding stress and inflammation to it) without the benefits of *really* exerting your body (inducing an adaptation and compensation to be stronger than before the exertion).

dedicated to Zone 2. Clint was harsh, but this is often how male friends show each other that they care; truth in love. I was indeed a downright fool and doing my body no favours.

At the time, it did not make sense to train at easy talking pace. Until I tried it. I started most of my training exercises in Zone 2, with a few Red Zone efforts. After months of employing this formula, I found that I improved. I became a better runner; leaner, faster, stronger. I started winning races again. More importantly, I started becoming healthier. I became more resilient to illness. I had more energy. I recovered faster. I realised that I had been missing out on these great side effects.

Be Patient (Or Become One)

Do you ever find that even though you are pushing yourself harder and harder every day, you do not see the results in races? The answer may be exactly this, that you are most likely at a Zone 3 plateau - as I was. You are possibly pushing too hard too often, and not running slow enough often enough, to recover.

The first rule is to keep your easy days extremely easy, and your hard days hard. What took me some time to grasp is that Zone 2 is even slower than the 'easy talking pace' that most training programs advocate. Using my heart rate monitor while running, even in Zone 3, I can speak and hold a conversation easily. Ideally you want to create a training program (or a way of life), that allows you to run easy days in Zone 2 to elicit a recovery response, increase aerobic capacity, and burn fat. An easy hour in Zone 2 will provide more benefit than a moderately hard paced effort for that same hour.

The important thing to understand here is this: 80-90% of our exercise should be done in this easy zone.

There are three reasons for this.

ONE, we do not want to add stress to our bodies.

TWO, we do not want to add inflammation to our bodies.

THREE, Neural Re-Education.

Some of you might still be wondering, "But how do I get faster?"

There is no other way to put this, when you train hard, you train *hard*. I mean throw-up intensity kind of hard. Provided you have done enough sessions the previous days in Zone 2 and your resting heart rate is low, that day is the perfect time to push a high heart rate.

In running circles, you would say on your hard training days: *Leave it all on the road.* Leave your blood, sweat and tears on the road. On these days you do not hold back. These days are where you stress the body enough to force the body into supercompensation, as described in previous chapters. The purpose of the 'hard' or 'red' days *is* to break the body down, provided you allow for adequate recovery of course. At this stage, Zone 2 running will promote the much-needed recovery. There is no major benefit to be gained from *just* outside of Zone 2 when you could be doing Red Zone efforts.

Happy Medium

If you are still uncertain when to train in Zone 2, a practical way to implement this system of training is to throw away your 'everyday pace[139]' mentality. It is this pace that leads you into a hard run at the huge cost of recovery and body adaptation.

You determine when to undertake Zone 2 recovery days by

---

[139] *Just* outside of Zone 2. Historically known as Zone 3 or the Orange Zone. The Voldemort of running paces. The pace that shall not be run. The pace that, hopefully by the end of this chapter and book, you never visit again. Too much Zone 3 running is the gateway drug to overuse injuries, loss of motivation and potential pain.

eliciting your resting heart rate and checking it every morning to see if you have recovered enough to do higher Red Zone intensity. This method is called Heart Rate Variability training, and it has proven most valuable to me in preventing overtraining and avoiding illness and injury.

Listen to Your Body

Below are two pictures of my actual Garmin watch with the resting heart rate graph that I view every morning. It details a clear picture of what is happening with my body.

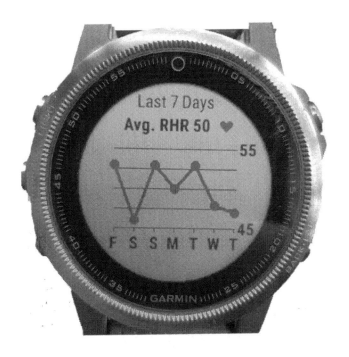

In the above picture, notice a few things.

Friday, I had a Zone 2 day because my heart rate was raised on Friday morning. Saturday, I woke up rested, and I ran a hard 25km long run. No matter who you are, except for Eliud or Mo, you will certainly feel a 25 km run the following day. Your legs will feel heavy. The result of this effort was a raised heart rate on Sunday morning, as expected. On Sunday I only stretched and went for an easy cycle. On Monday, I had clearly recovered, and at the time I was not working on Mondays and therefore could go for a long easy Zone 2 run. On Tuesday I had a raised heart rate[140]. Instead of training hard on this day, I had another Zone 2 recovery day. The result of the back-to-back Zone 2 days was obvious on Wednesday. My body was completely recovered. On Wednesday, I did a core session[141]. On Thursday, my body was completely recovered.

---

[140] Normally I would be rested after any easy Zone 2 day. Except on this Tuesday I was not properly recovered. Even though I woke up *feeling* fantastic, my body clearly had not recovered - based on my resting heart rate. Had I trained hard on this day, there is a strong likelihood I would have become sick or picked up an injury. This is *why* and *how* this system of training is so superior to any I have tried before.

[141] Remember the importance of core strengthening from Chapter 7. Core sessions include a range of Pilates- or Yoga- type of exercises. These include anything that promotes re-educating the body concerning what the core muscles are meant to do, as most of our *cores fall asleep* thanks to back rests and well marketed "lumbar supports".

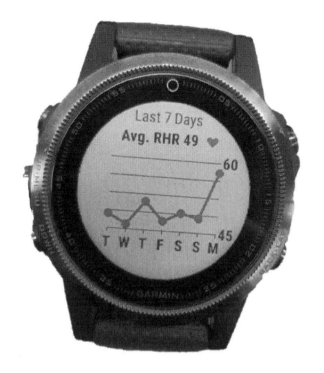

Take the picture above as another example; the week leading up to the London Duathlon. Wednesday was my last hard training session, and the heart rate showed it on Thursday morning by being slightly raised. Sunday was the race day, with maximum effort running and cycling for just over two hours, and the body felt it on Monday morning. The whole of the next week consisted of dedicated Zone 2 recovery days.

Professional vs Amateur Athletes

Now let me introduce you to Brad[142]. Even with his full-time job as a company director and his family schedule, he still has time to put in ten to fourteen training sessions a week. Most professional triathletes do the same number of training sessions as Brad. The only difference between their sessions and Brad's sessions is recovery time. While professional athletes may spend these days playing PlayStation, having a massage, and sleeping during the day, Brad and most other true amateur athletes are at work, where next to no recovery happens. It is safe to say that the only difference between Brad and a professional, is recovery hours.

Here are Brad's words, verbatim:

There are things that I have always felt amateurs lack compared to professionals. Recovery and sleep are the big ones. If I need to do a two-hour biking session, I need to wake up at 4:00 am to get it done before I do the school run and go to work. This is a definite compromise on sleep. Most of the time when you wake up at 4 am, you have normally done a session the night before, so the duration of your sleep is already limited. I compare myself to the professionals. They are getting their eight to nine hours regularly and are also power napping during the day. That is something I can never do. It is not a luxury I have.

So, when we speak about marginal gains, those small things make a massive difference, and realistically I cannot be getting up at 3:30 am and still expect to get any sort of respectable sleeping hours.

I think that is where most amateurs fall short - the recovery period directly after training, coupled with sleep deficiency. Recovery is key. Training breaks the muscles down; it is the

---

[142] Bradley Birkholtz. One of my training partners, fulltime businessman, great husband, and father, and one of the best age group triathletes in the world. Brad taught me to be diligent. I have never met a more dedicated person. Brad is proof that if you want to make time for something, *busy* is not an excuse.

recovery that makes you stronger. That is where I would love the opportunity to bank eight to nine hours every day and be able to bring myself down slowly after training. I am already pushing 18 to 22 hours a week of training. That is only five or six hours less than the professionals. It is the recovery where the professionals trump me.

Running vs Triathlon Injuries[143]

One last example of using this formula in sport and how effective it is in avoiding injuries is the incidence of overuse injuries in triathletes compared to runners. Overuse injuries drastically favour the latter. That is because even if a triathlete is fatigued in one discipline, for example running, he or she can still train hard in one of the other two disciplines the following day. Pure runners cannot train more than two days consecutively in the Red Zone without the strong likelihood of injuring themselves. I see that in practice every day.

By default, triathletes allow themselves to recover better as most are performing around three runs a week as opposed to six runs a week for runners. Cross training, as I discussed in the second chapter, is a vitally important part of running. And vice versa, running is strengthening for cycling and swimming.

Here is one last reason why cross training is a great idea: You are more likely to get more enjoyment out of training by virtue of different stimulations. I have tried it and I have

---

[143] Triathlon injuries. This is what I wrote my master's dissertation on. At the time, my supervisors recommended that I rather choose one of the three sports, as a masters in triathlon would mean reviewing all three sports. It would be too big they said. I fought it, and I paid the price. My dissertation was over 250 pages and took three months longer to finish. Looking back, this set me up to one day work alongside some of the greatest sportspersons on the planet. The moral of the story is: pick your battles and if you have the passion for something, go for it. Remember: a dream, with an achievable plan, becomes reality.

experienced both. Running six days a week eventually becomes monotonous. Even though I am not competing in triathlons currently, I train like a triathlete. By this I mean that I incorporate running, swimming, cycling, and the other pillars of MoveMed rehabilitation (core, flexibility, and proprioception) in my daily lifestyle.

Give it a try.

Point to ponder: Patience is a virtue, therefore learn to be patient, or become one.

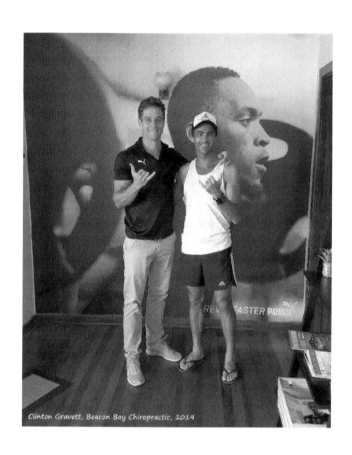

Clinton Gravett, Beacon Bay Chiropractic, 2019

13 : Move

Jon's Stress and inflammation profile: high.
Emotional stress high from working long
hours. Chemical stress, diet high in sugar,
refined foods. Physical stress of overtraining
coupled with lack of sleep and inadequate
recovery. *The room for improvement quite
frankly is huge (Donald Trump's voice).*

The benefits of exercise are compounding in nature,
like a cartoon snowball that gets bigger and more
impressive as it rolls down the hill. As you get fitter,
more flexible, stronger, etc., your body allows you to use a
greater proportion of the muscle, or more of the joint's range
of motion. This cycle continues, and what you put in; you get
out. The benefits are not only physical or visible, as you may
have grasped thus far.

These benefits apply to all of us, regardless of our
demographic, or fitness level. Hopefully by the end of this
book, or by the end of this chapter at least, you will understand
exercise in a different way to the dominant discussions

centered on losing weight, preventing disease and making our bodies look a certain way. Exercising could prolong your life. Whether you run, swim, dance, cycle, row, lift weights, do Yoga, Pilates, CrossFit, participate in team sports or even just stretch at home or walk around the block - it is worth your time and it is a good investment because movement *is* medicine. How so you ask?

Exercise does all kinds of things that a pill just cannot do. I have often wondered why it is not prescribed in the same way that a medication is. Exercise immediately releases endorphins and endocannabinoids, which instantly reduce pain, anxiety and produce a sense of ecstasy[144]. Fitness through physical exercise should be the number one prescription from a doctor, but it is not. There are various reasons for this: we have become accustomed to seeking relief from pain through over the counter and prescription medications rather than determining what is causing the pain in the first place. There is more money in prescribing drugs; shorter consultation times equate to even more money-generating consultations; and educating someone takes a whole heap of time and compassion energy without the financial rewards. Here are 19 reasons why I believe we should all exercise, why we should *move*. Some of these you would not have attributed to exercise and some you may know already.

ONE: Exercise creates anti-inflammatory responses

If you have been paying attention, you already know that to create a healing environment we are involved in a constant

---

[144] "Endo" means the body produces it. "Orphine" is from the word morphine - your body's homemade pain killer. "Cannabinoid" is from the word cannabis. *Marijuana.* Talk about getting high on your own supply. How incredible is the human body?

battle between stress and too much inflammation. In terms of decreasing inflammation, there are many biochemical reasons that show how low-grade exercise decreases inflammation, and I do not want to bore you with those. What I can share is what we have found in patients who do exercise.

I can confidently argue that low grade exercise, like Zone 2 running, produces an anti-inflammatory response.

Here is an example.

June 2018

Rust Cohle, a 45-year-old male patient presents at the practice. Patient claims that he is normally good at detecting when things are going wrong.

He presents with a previously diagnosed "ITB". (This is not a diagnosis. This is an abbreviation for a structure, the iliotibial band. The diagnosis should at least have been ITBS - Iliotibial Band Syndrome, which is still a very lazy diagnosis). The patient explains that he has tried everything but this ITB will not go away. He has even tried resting it. He explains that he has now resorted to running anyway, until he needs an operation.

We rule out Baker's cysts and Codman's tumours. Both sound like products from food producers but they are not[145].

Diagnosis is chronic lateral collateral ligament strain as a result of the fact that Rust was exercising too hard and not recovering (Zone 3 training increases inflammation in the injury).

Rust responded to a NRE protocol and training modification to incorporate more low-grade Zone 2 exercise.

---

[145] Baker's cysts are fluid-filled sacs that form in the back of the knee and are associated with degenerative conditions of the knee. Codman's tumour is another name for a chondroblastoma, which is an extremely rare bone tumour. Under a microscope, this tumour has a chicken-wire pattern of calcification.

Over a two-week period, his pain disappeared, and after six weeks he surpassed all other outcome measures[146].

Firstly, the good-to-knows:

ONE. If you have ever been diagnosed with "ITB", ask the diagnosing person what exactly is wrong with the band. Is it inflamed, torn, strained, compensating for a dodgy hip? Have they ruled out meniscus, ligamentous and stress fracture possibilities? You get the idea.

TWO. Rest alone is not treatment. *Active rest* is. You need to be helping the body recover with other interventions such as heat, ice, stretching, and treatment, of course. Rest will prevent something from getting worse, sure, but it very often will not be enough on its own.

THREE. We make these observations on a weekly basis. The only conclusion we can infer is that low grade exercise has anti-inflammation properties and Neural Re-Education is essential to improve injuries in the long-term.

TWO: Exercise improves resistance to stress

Regularly breaking the stress (cortisol) cycle is extremely important. There are many ways to do this, but I find the most effective is doing exercise. Remember, cortisol breaks the body down, and is released when we are stressed. The body will take some time to start secreting cortisol again once this stressed state has been broken.

When you exercise, your body produces many things. One of these things is endorphins, which are your body's natural doses of morphine. You feel better because there is less cortisol or stress hormone. Remember that we are not designed

---

[146] Outcome measures are important milestone tests that we conduct with patients every four to six weeks to gauge how they are responding to treatment. The minute that they stop showing improvements, I have either missed something, (and we reassess and change the plan accordingly), or I refer.

for chronic stress (and I think it is fair to say that the global biomedical fraternity would agree on this). Rather, we are designed to chase animals and rest - that is to say, experience acute stress, followed by recovery.

THREE: Exercise provides pain relief

The right kind of exercise will help relieve your pain.

Many of the pain-relieving drugs people take work on receptors for chemicals that the body is designed to produce. When you exercise, you produce most of those chemicals. The chemicals are there, not only to make you feel good, but to relax you, to make you feel better, and thereby to decrease your stress and cortisol. Remember, chronic stress is toxic.

Your body makes its own 'cannabis' during exercise. The "runner's high", usually attributed to endorphins, is likely caused by endocannabinoids.

Remember that pain, which is the main symptom that causes people to seek medical advice, is often the last to present and the first to go away. It is a poor indicator of wear and tear. Better symptoms to listen to (and which would warrant a check) are mundane things like stiffness, fatigue, irritability, headaches and odd sensations down your arms or legs. I have found that these are more accurate than pain in terms of finding areas of dysfunction.

FOUR: Exercise prevents obesity

Exercise helps your body use up excess energy stores known as fat cells or adipose tissue.

FIVE: Exercise could prevent surgery

It would possibly cause arthritis in my own hands if I had to write about every patient for whom we were able to prevent surgery (or for whom we were able to prolong functional years). Seeing somebody's face when you tell them that they do not need surgery anymore is pure job satisfaction. By way of demonstration, here is just one example.

September 2014

Dexter Morgan, a 27-year-old male patient presents to the practice. Patient explains that he has a killer pain in his hip.

Dexter has a history of competitive power lifting and water polo and has developed hip pain that was excruciating and waking him up at night. Patient was assessed by the top orthopaedic surgeon in his city, in South Africa, and to quote Dexter, the surgeon had told him, "you will be the youngest hip replacement I have performed".

We rule out Nelson's Syndrome. Which has nothing to do with Nelson Mandela[147].

Diagnosis is chronic bursitis of his left hip because of overuse (simple hip problem that is easy to treat conservatively).

Dexter chooses to avoid surgery and decides to take up running (which is the polar opposite to power lifting and at the time, in 2014, this was not my immediate recommendation).

---

[147] Nelson's syndrome is a rare clinical manifestation that occurs in up to 47% of patients as a complication of removing both adrenal glands, a procedure that is used to control Cushing's syndrome in patients with Cushing's disease. It is interesting to note that Cushing's syndrome is a condition caused by having too much cortisol in your body. Cortisol is the same hormone that your body produces during stress, remember. Common symptoms of Cushing's syndrome include more body fat on your chest, tummy, neck or shoulders. Your face may also be red and puffy.

Six years later, Dexter has completed ten road running marathons and an ultramarathon (56km). He has not been to see the orthopaedic surgeon again.

The good-to-knows:

ONE. Get a second opinion. Not only is my brother an orthopaedic surgeon, but I have referred hundreds of patients directly for surgery. If the joint is not completely wrecked, it *may* respond to conservative treatment.

TWO. I played a minimal role in this case. The patient made a choice to change. The patient made a choice to not be defined by a diagnosis. This patient taught me the power of exercise and the power of conscious decisions.

THREE. Again, we see that Zone 2 exercise has anti-inflammatory properties and we can conclude that it is possible to physically reconstruct a joint if you are prepared to put in the time. Remember the concept *change is inevitable.*

SIX: Autophagy

Autophagy is the body's way of cleaning out damaged cells, to regenerate newer, healthier cells. "Auto" means *self* and "phagy" means *eat*. Yes, you can actually train your body to eat itself, and yes, sometimes you want it to.

This is because autophagy is an evolutionary self-preservation instrument through which the body can remove damaged cells (cancer cells are an example) and recycle parts of them toward cellular repair and cleaning. Another way of starting this self-eating process is with intermittent fasting, but we will see more on this later in the book.

SEVEN: Exercise reduces blood pressure and risk of Type 2 Diabetes

Chronic hypertension is the most basic form of heart disease and it can easily be understood by anyone: increase the pressure in your blood vessels and your heart will need to pump harder than it needs to.

One of the causes of hypertension is plaque formation in the arteries that builds up from consuming certain fats through one's diet. Exercise helps reduce your blood pressure, in part, by stimulating the body to burn more fat for energy.

Type 2 diabetes is slowly becoming a world-wide public health problem. Even if you do not care about the health of the world, you should care about your own risk of diabetes. The difficulties of adult-onset Type 2 diabetes pose a serious risk to your physical wellness and health. By engaging in regular physical exercise, you improve your body's ability to metabolize glucose, the key to staving off this disease.

EIGHT: Exercise bolsters your immune system

Exercise makes you less vulnerable to falling ill from viruses that cause Colds or Flu symptoms. On the other hand, too much exercise and not enough recovery, will of course lower your immune system.

NINE: Exercise keeps your bones strong

Another normal age-related change in life is the loss of bone mineral strength, which can often develop into Osteoporosis. Exercise, particularly resistance training with weights or running, helps maintain your bone health.

Have you ever thought about how a broken leg heals in six weeks? Or how a broken collarbone sometimes does not heal?

The impact of weight going through a bone is what stimulates growth, that is why sometimes a collarbone will not fuse properly (or at all), as there is not much weight going *through* it. This is how weightbearing exercise keeps your bones strong, by constantly stimulating growth and repair[148].

TEN: Exercise improves breathing

Exercise improves how you breathe, both in terms of efficiency, (the stronger your breathing muscles are, the less energy they need to physically open and close your chest cavity during breathing), and efficacy (your body has the potential to deliver more oxygen per breath).

As we grow older, the trend is for our bodies to gradually grow weaker. Aging changes lung tissue in some ways that cannot be changed by exercise. The good news is that exercise can drastically improve your breathing. You may have noticed that non-exercisers will have to regularly catch their breath on escalators and lifts and after leaving their desk for a coffee break.

ELEVEN: Exercise boosts energy and suppresses your appetite

A strange spinoff perhaps, but the more exercise I do, the healthier I want to eat and the more energy I have. Of course, I am speaking about moderate Zone 2 exercise. Following a hard day of training in the Red Zone, my appetite increases, and my energy decreases until my body has recovered.

---

[148] Yes, before you say it, too much weightbearing is not a good thing either. The main reason being that overtraining will decrease recovery time. This, in turn, will weaken your bones. Perform some weight bearing exercise, then return to Zone 2 for the recovery.

With exercise, your body begins functioning more efficiently and therefore you have more oxygen to fuel your body's cells. As a result, you can go about your daily activities feeling less fatigued, less stressed, and less exhausted.

Fake it until you make it. Although exercising early in the morning or late in the afternoon may feel literally like the last thing you have the energy to do, force it a few times and eventually your body will crave the feeling of extra energy and all the other benefits discussed in this chapter. This craving happens subconsciously. The 'Fake-it' stage usually lasts three weeks, after which the faking is not needed anymore.

No matter how convincing I am in explaining this to patients, only those who make the choice of starting will experience it.

TWELVE: Exercise reduces the risk of arthritis

The management of arthritis is more effective than the internet tells you. Arthritis is one of the most experienced chronic illnesses in middle-aged to older patients. It occurs due to abnormalities in the cartilage and osteophytes (which are bony spikes or lips that form around the joints).

Unlike the other physical benefits of exercise, reducing the chances of arthritis does not depend on heavy duty aerobic activity or even weight training. In fact, you may heighten your risk of arthritis if you do too much of the wrong kind of exercise. Zone 3 and harder running efforts can cause you to be more likely to develop arthritis, since these stressors tilt your healing seesaw in favor of aggravation.

Engaging in stretching and flexibility training through Yoga, Pilates, or other ways to increase the range of movement of your joints, reduces the risk of arthritis. Proprioception of course, will also be beneficial as it will lower your risk of injury through muscle tears or torn ligaments, and in the process protect your joints from damage caused by overuse.

THIRTEEN: Exercise improves your sex life and self-confidence

I am aware that this may or may not apply to you, and that one's sex life and self-confidence may or may not be related to each other, however, if this is the one and only reason that motivates you to start exercising, it remains a good one. You could call it 'Sexercise'.

I recall a patient of mine from a few years ago. The guy was in impressive physical form; I mean you could grate cheese on his six-pack. I asked him what he was training for; was it body building or fitness modelling? (These are the common answers nowadays.) His answer was sublime: "To look good naked." Fair enough!

Regarding your sexual performance, there is a physical aspect to the act. Moderate and consistent exercise is likely to make you *feel* more fit and be more fit, which in turn will benefit your interest in and ability to carry out sexual activity. It is a win-win really.

Feeling healthy and feeling good about ourselves is linked in many ways to our self-confidence, which can translate into the way we engage with our sexuality, and the way we express it.

FOURTEEN: Exercise helps you sleep better

We know, from the chapter on *Recovery, Sleep and Off-seasons,* that sleep is one of the fundamentals of true recovery. I can recall countless nights when I either battled to fall asleep or had disrupted sleep. I rationalised this by thinking I had not burned enough energy compared with my energy intake. My body, therefore, was battling to rest because it had excess energy. And this is often the case.

243

A stressed body will physically hamper your ability to rest as it is still in its "fight or flight" mode. As mentioned previously, exercise counteracts the stress cycle. Purely being less in this state will allow you to sleep better.

FIFTEEN: Exercise lowers tendencies towards anxiety and depression

When you exercise, you redeploy your attention from your daily problems to the act of exercise. I find that I can gain a new perspective on even the most troubling concerns in my life by taking an exercise break. As your levels of endorphins increase, your feelings of worry also start to diminish. When you return to these daily problems, you can approach them with transformed energy, and a fresh perspective.

One example was the first SMILE[149] study in 2012. Duke University performed this study on 156 patients divided into three groups: one group was on Zoloft[150], another was on exercise alone and the third group was on a combination of exercise and medication. The exercise was walking or jogging at 70-80% of their maximum heart rate (around Zone 2 - who would have guessed that?), for 30 minutes, three times a week.

The study revealed that exercise is *as* effective as medication in reducing depression in patients and that exercise may reduce the risk of depression relapse.

---

[149] Standard Medical Intervention versus Long-term Exercise. I cannot even make this kind of research up. It is just so interesting that you do not see this information exploited in mainstream media or on television – what am I missing?

[150] Sertraline, sold under the brand name Zoloft among others, is an antidepressant. Common side effects include diarrhea, sexual dysfunction, and troubles with sleep. Serious side effects include an increased risk of suicide in those less than 25 years old. Yip, personally, I would at least try exercise before taking this.

No harm, no foul, right? Why would you not choose exercise over prescription drugs if you could? There are no major side effects, and you can change the chemistry in your brain in some incredible way.

Let me be straight about this - depression and depressive people are two different things.

Depression, when diagnosed correctly as a chemical imbalance, is an illness. Obviously, exercise alone will not cure this, but I believe it could be a beneficial supplement to prescription medication.

I am speaking to the many people who have been put onto antidepressant medications merely for symptoms of depression when they most likely suffer from chronic stress. I reckon exercise is a better alternative to prescription drugs in most of these cases.

SIXTEEN: Exercise is fun

For me, exercise is a way of life. Of course, not everyone will find the same joy in sweating as I do, in the same way as I do not understand how some people love shopping and find solace in 'Retail Therapy'. However, I do urge everyone to give themselves the chance to enjoy exercise because the positive effects are immense.

If you find the kind of exercise that fits your personality and motivational needs, you can have a good time while your body does the work. Whatever your exercise preference is, once you get into a routine, you will find that the activity itself becomes rewarding.

SEVENTEEN: Exercise could make you clever

Exercise (and particularly resistance training) is beneficial for improvements of, on average, over 10% in cognitive function, memory, and executive functions (things like problem-solving and decision-making) among elderly people. These functions are necessary for independent living and are affected by conditions such as Alzheimer's disease and other types of dementias.

Until now, neuroplasticity[151] was thought to cease by the age of five. It has now been found that this is not the case, and that fitness training has been shown to induce neuroplasticity even in the elderly.

You do not even have to exert yourself that much to experience a memory boost; moderate walking can help your brain's memory center, the hippocampus, maintain its health and vitality. Preserving the neurons in your brain may prevent or delay the onset of Alzheimer's disease.

EIGHTEEN: Exercise controls addiction

Exercise may help you stop smoking, taking stimulants or drinking too much alcohol.

This goes hand in hand with reason number three. Exercise itself is like a drug. It can be as addictive as any other substance or habit you have developed over time. The only exception is that this addiction could save you from all types of harmful addictions. While you are exercising, your brain releases a brain chemical called Dopamine which influences the pleasure-reward area of the brain. Our cravings for food, drug, sex, and alcohol are formed as a result of Dopamine imbalances in the brain, and exercise aids in balancing these levels.

---

[151] The ability of your brain to physically grow and develop new neural connections. Most neuroplasticity happens before the age of five, but it never stops. For this reason, invest in the most nutritious food for your children. You will see later how clean eating promotes regeneration.

NINETEEN: Exercise saves you money

Most exercise activities are a fun way to spend and end your day, without costing you money. For example, going for a hike, walking, or cycling, are far cheaper than an afternoon spent drinking in a pub, and much better for your health.

Free exercise is of course also cheaper than any medication or pill, and if that pill is not essential for your survival, exercise may be one of the catalysts that free you from your dependence on it.

If you were to meet any of my headache patients, you would see this. They have endured an almost lifelong dependence on medications, but with some treatment, and more importantly, the incorporation of exercise into their lives, their dependence on medications for their headaches normally disappears.

Exercise can tilt the health equation back in your favour, you just need to *move*.

Point to ponder: Exercise does all kinds of things that a pill just cannot do.

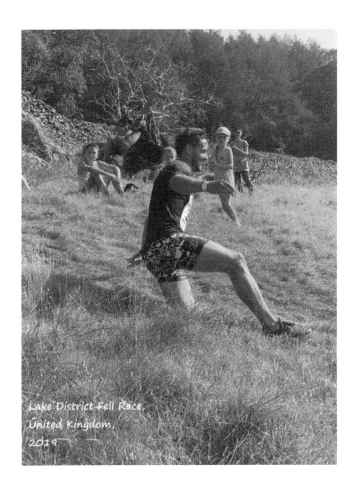

Lake District Fell Race,
United Kingdom,
2019

14 : Your First Time

Jon's orthopaedic examination findings:
Bechterew's, Slump 8 and Kemp's tests all
positive on the Right. Lesegue's and
Braggard's signs on the right. Minor's sign on
the left. At least we now know what is wrong.

Y ou often hear that your first time is the most memorable. You are likely to feel vulnerable, sometimes awkward, you could both be nervous, unsure of what happens next or you may even feel some discomfort. Overall, your first time should be educational, at the very least, and having taken the right precautions, there should not be any unwelcome consequences.

When you see a practitioner, of any kind, for the first time, you will undergo a case history, a physical examination and most often a treatment (this could be a direct referral to someone else if the condition is not in the scope of practice).

First impressions are important, so my mantra is always; Display confidence, smile, make eye contact and be honest.

Part One: The Case History

Flipping through the health questionnaire first-time patients complete upon arrival, I am looking for a starting point - what are the events, experiences, routines, habits, choices, that have collided to bring you here. Have you seen a Chiropractor before? What is the main complaint? Oh, I see you suffer from depression too. We will investigate that diagnosis. Interesting. You have ticked the box that indicates you would like corrective care. This is a great start. I can work with that[152].

Good day Mrs Granger.

Hi Dr Coetzee.

Cannot stop my mind wondering about humorous Harry Potter references!

We shake hands.

You can tell a whole lot about a patient in a handshake and through eye contact. Weak hands indicate maybe C6 neurological deficit or social insecurities. The patient cannot make eye contact - Horner's syndrome or social insecurities, low self-esteem. Cold hands - either Raynaud's disease or it is just cold outside.

Please take a seat.

I watch the demeanour of the patient. How well they carry themselves speaks into their psyche and I also note antalgic gait patterns (foot drop / steppage gait indicates deep peroneal nerve and L5 issues, pain gait we think arthritis, choreiform gait we think Huntington's Disease, ataxic gait we think alcohol abuse and sensory gait we think diabetes). Do they slouch in the chair? It may possibly be the result of postural muscle memory.

How can I help you?

---

[152] Recent research on patient compliance stated that upward of 40% of patients are "useless" at doing what you advise them. We are advised to underestimate patient compliance but to overemphasize it anyway. I prefer to overestimate my patients.

252

I have this pain in my back. Lower back.

Okay, and whom have you seen for it?

Oh, I have been everywhere. I have tried everything. And I am so over being prescribed anti-inflammatories and pain killers. They only help temporarily.

Clearly, the patient has not been given a proper diagnosis yet. This patient has not been educated about why they are on medication or what else they could try for their ailment. If conservative treatment fails over six weeks, including my treatment plan, I am meant to refer the patient as soon as possible. Diagnosis and management 101 - or it should be. I always start with SOCRATES[153].

Where exactly is the pain? Can you point to it?

It is here (patient points to her left sacroiliac joint) and goes to here (hand moves into left buttock) and sometimes into the leg (left). Also, across my whole back sometimes.

When did it start?

It is important here to ascertain when the first ever back symptom happened, and stiffness is indeed a symptom. Also, it is necessary to establish when the recent episode of pain started. Usually for five to ten years patients have experienced stiffness or the odd niggle. Recent onset is anything from same day to two months.

Five years ago, when I started my desk job. Recently it flared up after a trip to Europe to our family beach house.

That sounds posh[154]. Granger's spine has had more than five years of abnormal postures and stressors. A sitting job has

---

153 SOCRATES is a mnemonic acronym used to evaluate the nature of pain that a patient is experiencing. Site, Onset, Character, Radiation, Alleviating factors, Timing, Exacerbating factors, Severity (1-10).

154 I only recently learnt that 'POSH' is actually an acronym for "port out, starboard home", describing the north-facing cabins taken by the richest passengers travelling from Britain to India and back. Only the wealthy could afford these cabins. I am not sure where the posh accent comes from though, probably all the gap *yaahs* (years).

a whole set of its own stressors. The fact that a different bed, pillow and travelling flared it up means it was on the verge of a flare-up anyway.

What is the pain like? An ache? Stabbing?

It is a dull ache across the lower back, occasional sharp pain in the dimple and the leg pain is more of a numbing pins and needles type of pain.

Dull achy pain - I am thinking long-term low-grade muscle spasm in the quadratus lumborum muscles, most likely due to inactive core muscles or purely compensation for the forward bending during all those years of desk work, as the muscles try to extend the flexing spine. Occasional sharp pain in the dimple? Most likely a sacroiliac joint strain, as the body is compensating to take pressure off the primary lesion, TBD (to be diagnosed). When a patient explains anything related to numbness, tingling, burning, shooting, or electric pain, alarm bells must go off. This means a nerve is being irritated and needs to be diagnosed as soon as possible.

Any other signs or symptoms associated with the pain?

Not really. Some bloating maybe. Some heartburn every now and then.

Things just became interesting. Bloating, rule out a typical average diet, white carbs maybe? Dairy? Maybe general nerve tension from the chronic back tension, affecting signals to the gut. Heartburn? Rule out vagus nerve irritation. Heartburn is often caused by loss of tone in the oesophagus sphincter[155], which can be relieved by adjusting the upper cervical joints, and restricted joints in the neck and mid back.

In the mornings I take a while to get moving. It is painful in the lower back dimple. The dull ache is always there. And the leg numbness is felt as soon as I sit or drive.

It seems we have at least three mechanical issues here now.

---

[155] If the muscle that needs to contract to keep acid in your stomach loses some of its tone, then acid could enter the oesophagus causing heartburn.

Morning pain - I am thinking sacroiliitis[156]. Inflamed joints are always worse in the morning as the inflammation exudate settles inside the joint overnight, and as you wake up the first few compressions of the joint will be painful. Once the inflammation is moving again, it is not too bad. The long-term dull ache? I am still thinking spasm, or also low-grade inflammation in the lumbar joints in general. The nerve symptom of numbness which is made worse by sitting - I need to rule out discs. Discs compress with flexion compression forces, in other words when the patient bends forwards.

Does anything make the pain better or worse?

Lying down flat on my back helps. Heat helps. Massages makes things worse.

Ding! Ding! Ding! Jackpot. Lying down mechanically takes pressure off the joints, muscles and discs - this will help alleviate the pain. Heat application that helps the pain indicates to me that there is a protective muscle spasm. This kind of spasm is the body's natural compensation. However, it is the worst for the body long term as it prevents movement, and therefore prevents blood flow. Heat application increases blood flow and will reduce inflammation, a double whammy. You are probably wondering why it is a good thing if a massage makes things worse. It is because a massage will release the muscle tension that is protecting the back, and then the body is able to feel all the inflammation, joints or discs that are symptomatic. The body is clever like that, but it is also its own worst enemy. (Refer to the importance of NRE from the earlier chapters.)

How bad is the pain? 0 being no pain, 10 is excruciating pain.

A constant 2 but can reach a solid 7 during the worst flare-

---

156 Add 'itis' to the end of any word and that means its inflamed. Arthritis, inflamed joint. Sinusitis, inflamed sinus. Appendicitis, inflamed appendix. Vaginitis, run. Adding 'itis' to the end of a word is different to adding 'itus', as in pruritus ani, meaning itchy bum.

ups.

That is about right. 2 out of 10 is mild enough to live with, but bad enough to cause all sorts of long-term mechanical problems as we can clearly see[157].

Any other complaints? Neck pain? Midback pain? Headaches?

No neck issues. Only the odd headache.

How often do you get headaches? Daily? Weekly? Monthly? Back of the head, top, frontal, jaw or behind the eyes?

They are frontal and occur only maybe once or twice a month.

Bank this information for later, we know the main complaint is lower back and clearly neurological - which is urgent. But we know with nerve issues there are often other nerve tensions elsewhere in the spine.

It is from here that we develop a holistic view of our patient. Get to know the ins, outs and inside outs of the patient, their family history and lifestyle. Things like travel history, how their pain effects their lives, a full system review and psychosocial status.

What exercise do you do?

I am scared that exercise will make things worse. But I desperately want to exercise again because my depression has become worse since I stopped exercising.

Well Granger you have just become one of my favourite patients. You want to get better.

Do you smoke?

No.

Great. Research has now linked smoking directly with low back pain and also with erectile dysfunction. This is always a

---

[157] I believe, and it has been made very real in my practice, that 99% of the diagnosis is made from a proper case history. The physical examination should be confirming your differentials and obviously getting an understanding of the patient's physical health at present.

good time to consider stopping if you are male, and you smoke.

Do you have a family history of low back pain?

Dad had a disc operation a few years ago. I am not sure about Mom. We lived with Dad.

Cool. So genetically maybe a cartilage weakness, or Dad was just offered an operation before being given other options for disc treatments. "Lived with Dad." Okay, there may be a story here to link to depression. I must still probe this later.

Now your drug history - your medications I mean?

I need to know all the medications that a patient takes, as side effects from medications could be altering our diagnostic picture. Also, side effects from medications can be overly aggressive. Antibiotics increase chances of tendonitis issues. Statins cause muscle pain. Some are just poison. (For each medication ask them to specify: Dose, frequency, route and compliance[158].)

I take an antidepressant every day.

There it is.

You mentioned in your paperwork that you are depressed or have been diagnosed with that and you are on medication for that. Is that right?

Yes.

I am sorry to hear that. May I ask who diagnosed that and what the process was that they used to reach that diagnosis?

It was my GP. And he prescribed the antidepressants.

Were blood tests done? A psychiatrist consultation?

No.

Granger has been given a mind-altering and sometimes addictive medication, based on the reported symptom of a depressive person. And these medications are not from a specialist specializing in depression. No blood tests were done and therefore the opportunity to locate a potential external

---

158 Remember, 40% of patients display "useless" compliance. Therefore, we can assume the patient has not taken his/her medication as per the dosage and frequency, until proven otherwise.

cause that can be managed. I will encourage Granger to seek a second opinion for her medicated depression.

Would you like to be off those medications eventually?

Hell yes.

Hells yeah!

And what kind of work do you do? You mentioned desk work.

Yes, I am in banking.

Along with half of the London population, it seems.

Do you use a laptop or PC?

PC.

This is great, as lifting a desktop screen higher is golden for your siting posture. Actually, just a change of workstation is beneficial to try break some of the negative physical memory of someone's work environment.

Would you be able to get a standing desk?

Maybe.

Standing desks are 100-fold better for your spine than sitting. But you need to be careful not to go from sitting eight hours a day to standing for eight. It is too much, and you will experience agonizing back pain. Start with one hour a day standing for the first week and add another hour each week. Over two months you will be comfortable with standing.

Great, if I could write a motivation letter to your HR team to help get that ball rolling, please let me know.

What are your bed and pillow like?

I use a feather pillow, sometimes two.

Horrible.

Feather pillows are not the best. For your next birthday or Christmas, get yourself an orthopaedic memory foam pillow. It is essential to have the same support for your neck every night. Your body gets used to the support and the joints and muscles can rest overnight. That is why your neck and back often get stiff during or after holidays. A few nights with your neck in a different position can cause havoc. Imagine your neck is abnormally bent during your night's sleep. The joints compress on the inside of the curve and the ligaments and muscles stretch on the outside. All of these can cause irritation, inflammation and compensatory muscle spasm. Your classic *stiff neck* from travelling.

Do you sleep well? And how many hours a night do you get? Does your back ever wake you up at night?

I sleep okay, maybe like six hours a night. My pain does not wake me up. It did five years ago when it first started.

Six hours is not enough.

Something to take from this patient was that when we asked about history of trauma for a second time, she had completely forgotten about a fall through a roof, landing on her back and being knocked out.

It is unbelievable how the body and mind will often shut out major traumas. A few weeks ago, I ended up X-raying a patient and finding that they had a vertebra that was slipping forwards on the vertebra below it[159]. It was stable and had healed that way. This condition is either genetic or can be from trauma. The patient had confirmed that she had no previous traumas, but I probed further to be sure. It turned out she had been hit by a bus. No X-rays were taken of the lower back because she had suffered a head injury and the emergency team had focussed on that. This happens often. It is nobody's fault. The body will naturally block out old traumas - physical and emotional ones.

Any bruise means rupture of tissue - muscle, ligament, tendon, or joint most commonly. That bruise will heal with a heap of scar tissue, and if the patient does not have or is not

---

159 This means the patient has a broken back. Technically. It is called a *degenerative spondylolisthesis*. The little bones that join the front to the back of the vertebrae have broken away from each other. The medical term is *stress fractured*. Most of these *broken backs* we see in practice are caused by years of bad posture. The spine literally slowly breaks as a result of years of tension. That is where the word stress fracture comes from.

educated about the need for NRE after a trauma like that, scar tissue will form in abnormal planes of movement. He/she will have a massive mechanical risk for injuries in the future. Case in point.

In the magical case of Mrs Granger, a disc bulge is jumping out at me. L4/5. And at the same time, chicken or egg situation, (but less urgent), is the left sacroiliac joint strain and chronic quadratus lumborum myofascial pain and dysfunction. Headaches are most likely as a result of trigger points in the neck muscles.

Part Two: The Physical Examination

I always choose to perform the neurological part of a physical exam first. I will often explain to a patient that with great reflexes comes great response-ability.

It gets a laugh a third of the time. My jokes are generally rather lame or only funny to my outlandish sense of humour, and more often than not there is a tough audience. It turns out people in pain have often lost their sense of humour.

In Granger's case, we found massively diminished reflexes on the left leg, with loss of sensation in the outside of the shin. Luckily, there was no muscle weakness. Muscle weakness in my opinion is more of a red flag than the other peripheral nerve symptoms. If a muscle wastes away from nerve damage, that muscle will be permanently damaged. I have found that the other nerve symptoms can recover more easily. There was also a very subtle weakness in the right bicep reflex.

Now the diagnostic picture is looking like a clearly painted Monet.

There were positive orthopaedic tests for sacroiliac joint dysfunction, L4/5 and C0/C1 and C5/C6 in the neck. Granger also showed gross loss of range of motion in the lower back and neck. Remember, there was no neck complaint. The only hint of neck issues on history were heartburn and occasional frontal headaches.

The rest of the physical examination was unremarkable. There were trigger points in the lower back and gluteal muscles, and the trapezius in the neck, but none were reproducing the pain that the patient experienced. I was shocked that we could not reproduce the headaches. It was therefore a case that clinically warranted X-rays.

X-rays showed significant disc height loss L4/5 and C5/6, with severe degenerative changes C1/2.

The X-rays rarely surprise us. There are obviously exceptions, but 99% of the time, whatever changes are happening in the lumbar spine are also happening in the neck, and Granger was the perfect example.

Our original list of possible diagnoses was not far off. Disc bulge L4/5, left sacroiliac joint strain and chronic quadratus lumborum myofascial pain and dysfunction. Until the physical and X-rays were conducted, our headache cause was substantially off target. That is the beauty of the working progress of a systematic approach. Imagine if I had just treated the neck muscles in Mrs Granger's case? No wonder she had been everywhere, and nothing was helping. Medication will not fix mechanics, and physically treating the incorrect structure will be as useless.

The good-to-knows:

ONE. Remember your traumas. When I ask you for them, make sure you know them. They are so important for the state of your spine and nervous system.

TWO. If you can recall a trauma of some kind, no matter how insignificant it seems, ask yourself if it was accurately assessed at the time, and if adequate *Neural Re-Education* occurred. Granger had no real neck symptoms, yet the disc in her neck was non-existent from years of wear and tear on a damaged disc. Add a few years on to this, and when she turns 50 she will have severe disc degeneration in a few levels if she does not change the current stressors.

THREE. You have the right to ask questions. You should

be satisfied with the education you receive from your practitioner. *Doctor means teacher.*

FOUR. Post-consultation, if you have not seen a significant window of relief in six weeks, something is wrong. The initial diagnosis was incorrect, or if the practitioner is confident the diagnosis was correct, you need to be referred.

FIVE. Do not accept any diagnosis unless you have had all your concerns answered.

SIX. Do not accept life-changing diagnoses like depression lightly. Obtain a second and a third opinion if necessary and try conservative treatments for these before medications. There are numerous examples in this book.

Part Three: The Treatment

Mrs Granger underwent the six-week conservative trial and she responded incredibly well. She also opted to pay for a private MRI while we started treatment (MRI at the end of the chapter) which confirmed our diagnosis[160].

We continued to see longer windows of relief[161]. I now see her monthly for assessments and adjustments. It is a simple way to reduce the physical stress on her nervous system. She is on a core activation exercise program; she is running and

---

[160] It is great when this happens. Many patients question our diagnosis. Many patients tell me what they believe their diagnosis is after searching Google. I do not mind either of those, all it tells me is that the patient wants to get better. They have made a choice to find out more. And the first step of healing is always a conscious choice.

[161] Windows of relief. This is what you look for when you are treating someone for pain. If the patient describes moments or a few hours where they had no pain, or windows of relief, this is clinical gold. Windows means that for that specific time, there was no pain stimulus to the brain. Instead, there was a stimulus of normal function to the brain. The windows get longer and longer until they are permanent, provided the healing seesaw is in our favour - provided Neural Re-Education had been restored.

maintains her flexibility. She cleaned up her diet and prioritizes her recovery like sleep and Zone 2 exercise which further reduces chemical stress on her nervous system. She is now off her antidepressant medication, and there is less emotional stress on her entire body system.

The rewards are huge when the patient's ambition to get better matches my ambition to guide the healing process. The nervous system after all controls everything. It is time to make it a priority.

Mischief managed.

Point to ponder: The word doctor means teacher, therefore, have you been educated enough when seeing someone?

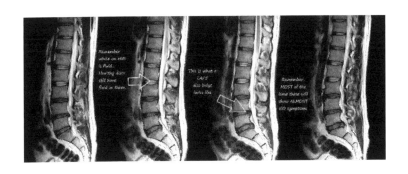

265

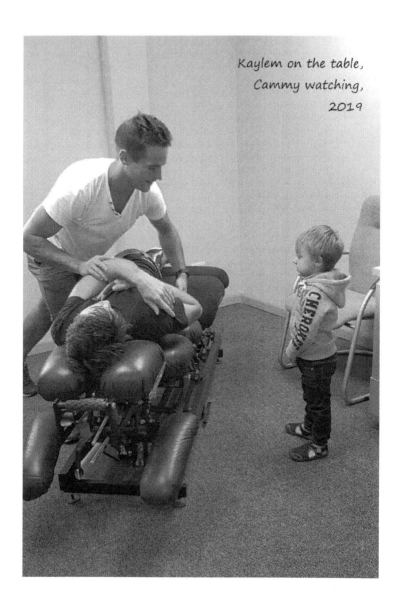

Kaylem on the table,
Cammy watching,
2019

15 : Headaches

Jon's knee orthopaedic examination findings: Tinel's Sign, Apley's Compression Test, Apley's Distraction Test and McMurray's Test all positive on the left medial knee. *It is pretty obvious what is wrong with his knee.*

I am proud to say that I was considered a nerd at school. As was my best mate Brett, whom I introduced earlier in the book. We were the most dedicated and enthusiastic members of our mathematics class. We just loved math! Now, I am not sure which I like more, mathematics or treating headaches. It is probably because they are so similar. It is about problem solving, and I find a natural satisfaction in solving any problem.

I understand that not all of us suffer from headaches, but we have all at least experienced the discomfort and inconvenience of one at some point or another and reached for the paracetamol to swat it away. Nevertheless, unpacking my favourite topic in this chapter will still be helpful for you as a reminder of what to do when the kraken arrives.

Besides being painful and annoying, headaches put you in a bad mood, and this is not good for relationships or any social interaction really. It is not good for energy levels. It is most certainly not good for productivity.

Here is the first math problem. How common are headaches?

Let us leave Google out of this one. It is my eighth year in private practice. On average, I have seen around sixty patients per week. The average work year consists of forty-eight weeks. I would guesstimate that every third patient I have seen comes in with a complaint of headaches, so roughly speaking, that makes around eight thousand headache treatments on average in a year. Suffice it to say, that headaches bad enough and frequent enough to seek treatment for, are pretty common.

If I were not bound by confidentiality laws, I could list all the patients, by name, whose headaches we could not diagnose or manage. For me this highlights the need for quality primary healthcare and education. Every structure mentioned in this chapter can be spatially summarized by placing the tip of your middle finger at the base of your head. Your finger would cover all the structures. Now if you push a little, you may feel tenderness. Let me explain.

By the nature of internal referrals, I understand that patients are likely to refer someone else to us that is struggling with the same health issue. We therefore attracted a great deal of headache patients, because as we helped more people with headaches, even more headache patients seemed to come seeking the same help.

The more exposure I had to headache sufferers and the various causal areas within their bodies, the more I was able to identify major areas not commonly treated in combination. In most cases, I found them related to the craniocervical junction, the area between the base of your skull and the first few vertebrae. It is an area so small it is almost impossible to give a definitive diagnosis based on feel alone, therefore symptoms, especially reproducible symptoms, are essential.

Typically, the patients suffering from headaches that I have treated have previously been diagnosed with migraines or tension headaches. Apparently, statistics show these to be the most common headaches. I am highly skeptical of these statistics because in my experience of asking patients how they were diagnosed, it seems that the method for diagnosing headaches is often done on case histories alone, and not by any manual examination.

Any diagnosis needs to be done systematically, like a mathematic algorithm, starting with a case history, physical examination, (both local and full body), to identify neuromusculoskeletal versus organ referral[162]. These findings need to be cross-referenced with the practitioner's clinical experience, research, and the psychosocial history of the patient.

Migraine patients tend to take a cocktail of medications when the headaches occur. A *migraine cocktail* is available for purchase over the counter at pharmacies in South Africa. I have also noticed that the majority of patients suffering from tension headaches are on anti-depressants. I mentioned a similar scenario with Mrs. Granger in the previous chapter, and the severity of the side effects of such medication, especially when patients are not clinically depressed. With simple mechanical treatment and rehabilitation exercises, we can generally have patients become less dependent on or completely off these medications.

It is simply a matter of old school diagnostics and new school treatments, which leaves me wondering why the medication-free and conservative option is not at least attempted before medication is prescribed?

---

[162] In other words, where exactly is the pain in your head coming from? Sounds like a question your doctor should be asking himself/herself. It seems that this rarely happens these days.

For years now, practices wherein I have worked have had the strangest business model. 'Fix' people as quickly as you can, treat them less and teach them what to do to prevent their coming back. The spinoff is that these patients refer their friends, their family, their colleagues or simply any acquaintance.

First, I work according to a key principle. If you can reproduce it, you can fix it. *Referred pain.* If one can add pressure to a structure in the neck, and it reproduces the same pain or symptom as the patient experiences during pathologic episodes, then, in my experience, we can manage it. And yes, sometimes the reproduced symptom or lack thereof means referring the patient pronto[163] and that is done quicker than you can phonetically pronounce Waldenstrom's macroglobulinemia.

---

[163] A quick sidenote. If you are reading this book, you are beyond privileged. If you disagree, then the mere fact that you can read puts you into a privileged class. Regarding headache treatment, you have seen in this book already how the health care systems currently in place often miss the boat completely. It is important to acknowledge here some of the other reasons why they are substandard. Take the NHS, and most government sponsored health care in other countries like SA, where health practitioners are trying to see as many people as possible with limited time and resources. My brother confirmed this for me. He works in a government hospital and can see 80 to 90 patients during one clinic day. Do the maths, there is only so much you can do in that time. Another aspect is that seeing a dietician, seeing a chiropractor, going to one's Yoga classes often seem to fall under the realm of the *wealthy* who have the time and the money to live such a 'pampered' life. Let us not beat around the bush here. Another facet to think about is that much of the working-class work 14 hours a day at a factory, or a warehouse, or as a labourer, and, purely due to time constraints, their health is not a priority. And when they experience pain, they need a quick fix to get back to work, especially the wage earners in countries like SA. So yes, I acknowledge all these things. *It is what it is*, but that is one of the reasons I wrote this book. To educate everyone and anyone about the benefits of preventing conditions like headaches and low back pain. And it should be evident now that movement is a great place to start.

If you have ever had physical treatment, you will have noticed that the therapist will push and prod their fingers directly into your injured and already painful body part, and they will have asked you if it was painful. There is method to this madness. What they are actually asking is, "Does that reproduce the pain you feel?"

If the answer is "No", that is most likely not the primary injury, and it is a compensation of sorts. We need to look elsewhere or refer the patient for further investigations.

If the answer is "Yes", this is a win.

Secondly, and particularly related to headaches, wherever a muscle refers pain, you can have dysfunction in that area. This is my hypothesis for a headache that is accompanied by blurred vision; if pain is referring behind the eye in the vicinity of the orbital muscles, (the muscles in your eye socket that move the eye and control the lens), you could have eye symptoms such as blurred vision, (if the lens cannot focus), or you could have eye twitches, (if the muscles of the eyelid spasm).

There is never a dull day in my line of work. I am always left wondering just how intricately and magnificently the body was designed in the first place.

Below is an example of what I call a 'textbook headache patient' of mine. The irony is that it seems no textbooks are used by some practitioners with regard to headache diagnosis.

June 2018

Michael Scott, a 43-year-old male patient, presents to the clinic. Patient explains that he runs an unorthodox office where he is the regional manager.

Patient describes long term headaches that he attributes to his posture at his desk, and stress. Michael describes a headache that starts at the base of his head, refers up the back of his head and around to behind his eyes. The pain behind his eyes can be one-sided, or on both sides, and it alternates, but more frequently it is left-sided. About a third of his headaches will be accompanied by dizziness and nausea, and every second month he has episodes of colds/flu and feels his sinus is blocked up. These episodes of flu are unaccompanied by fever.

We rule out Neck-tongue Syndrome, (which is not a type of foreplay), as well as a Thunderclap Headache, which actually is as scary as it sounds[164].

All other pertinent red flags are ruled out and we are left with a mechanical headache.

The patient describes his headaches, and we can categorize the different characteristics of the headache by what he has previously had done for them.

He describes the following:

PAIN BEHIND AND IN THE EYES. *He has had numerous unwarranted and costly eye tests and now uses prescription glasses because his headache was diagnosed as a headache from the eyes based on the location of the pain.*

PAIN AROUND THE FOREHEAD. *The patient recalls being prescribed antibiotics for his ongoing frontal sinus pain that was diagnosed as chronic sinusitis.*

PAIN AT THE BACK OF THE HEAD. *The patient has been told that he is stressed and now finds himself on antidepressant medication.*

Can we see the problem here? Let us carry on.

---

[164] Neck-tongue syndrome is characterized by pain at the back of the neck and numbness of the tongue lasting from just seconds up to one minute. It is caused by sudden movements of the head. I have seen a few of these in practice – fascinating. A Thunderclap headache is severe, sudden, explosive, unexpected and likened to a "clap of thunder". This headache could be associated with, (amongst many other causes), an unruptured aneurysm in your brain. *Red flag refer now!* I am eternally grateful that I have never seen one of these in practice before.

PAIN AT OR AROUND THE JAW. *The patient underwent corrective orthodontic work at the age of 30 to fix his jaw movement and biomechanics. However, he still experienced the same headaches after the procedures.*
A HEADACHE ASSOCIATED WITH NAUSEA. *The patient had frequently been diagnosed with migraines and finds himself reliant on cocktails of medications to help these headaches.*
A HEADACHE ASSOCIATED WITH DIZZINESS[165]. *The patient mentions a few prescriptions for antibiotics for middle ear infections that never resolved the headache or dizziness.*
A HEADACHE ASSOCIATED WITH CORYZA (COMMON COLD). *Do we need to go into what medications patients are given for apparent viral colds that would pass anyway, or that are not even viral infections in the first place?*

Cervicogenic Headache

Michael's headache was diagnosed as a cervicogenic headache ("Cervico" - meaning neck, "genic" meaning begins). We hypothesize that if the headache is a cervicogenic headache, then it should respond to treatment. The algorithm includes myofascial release of the SCM muscle and trapezius muscles. Also, part of this algorithm is adjustments - the physical act of getting the joints moving normally again.

Myofascial release is any technique the practitioner is comfortable with that will remove the trigger points in the muscle. The most effective I have found is dry needling,

---

[165] This symptom often does not present any pain. Often, I am treating a patient for low back pain, and it turns out, from their history, that they experience dizziness. This prompts us to investigate the neck simultaneously, and often we find similar, if not worse, degeneration in the neck, although the patient never had symptoms there. Remember, pain is a poor indicator of dysfunction. More on this later.

coupled with hard manual trigger-point therapy. Basically, this is where you push so hard into the muscle that the patient either screams at you or punches you. I have had both happen to me.

In Michael's case, he responds as expected. This raises a chicken or egg scenario: did the joint dysfunction cause the trigger points or did the muscle tension cause the joint dysfunction. If he had come to me ten years ago, we could have isolated which started first[166], but currently, the primary problem is a bit blurred and therefore we treat everything.

His pain is 80% improved after four treatments, and he further invests in his health by coming for a full Neural Re-Education protocol over six weeks. I now see him once a month and he experiences approximately six mild headaches a year now, most of which he can treat himself, at home, using heat and ice packs and stretching and exercise.

It is just math[167].

I would like to draw your attention to a few of the big guns in terms of headache causes. For all of them, we apply the algorithm above.

Pain: *If we can reproduce it, we can fix it.*

---

[166] And again, I acknowledge that *life happens* and many different circumstances (financial, family, physical distance, many others) prevent people from coming for regular screenings, and they wait for the pain to arrive. Often, the government institutions will not see you until your condition is really bad, and then they try put a band aid on the sinking ship. This is a common scenario for patients whom I see in practice. Patients have waited so long to get treatment that by the time they come in for an assessment, there are many areas to treat and these often overlap. For that reason, you should TRY to have regular physical screenings or consultations to essentially identify when the body is compensating for something and try to remove the stressors before they become symptomatic. Remember, pain is often the last symptom to show, and we forget that tension and muscle fatigue are symptoms that we overlook but which are so informative as to what is happening.

[167] Or it is just medicine.

Muscles

We know that muscles can cause pain, and more importantly can refer pain somewhere else. Medical doctors Travell and Simmons identified a phenomenon called a myofascial trigger point which is defined as a hyperirritable area inside a muscle that is associated with a tense band. You can feel these for yourself if you dig around in your neck using your finger.

Statistically it is highly unlikely your headache is caused by a brain tumour, and equally as rare as encephalitis, (your whole brain being inflamed). So, where do most muscular headaches originate from? More often than not, they are caused by myofascial trigger points in the neck or jaw muscles that refer pain over another muscle or area. Of course, it so much more intricate than that, and diagnoses involve a large chunk of tests (but this chapter is here to educate you about the big players in common headache causes).

SCM

Let us look, firstly, at the Sternocleidomastoid muscle[168]. This is the muscle that every vampire targets because of its close proximity to the carotid artery. This muscle was the main cause of Michael's headaches.

There are trigger points in this muscle, and if squeezed, they can refer pain around or behind the eyes, on the forehead over the eyes, at the back or top of the skull, across the cheek, and within the jaw.

In addition to the pain referral pattern and motor dysfunction, trigger points in this muscle can cause nausea,

---

[168] Have you ever wondered why some muscles have weird names? They are often from the original Latin words, or they are often the actual areas where the muscle attaches. So sternocleidomastoid, runs from the sternum or breastbone to the mastoid process at the base of the skull.

dizziness, coryza[169], and tearing (actual tears down your face) on the same side. That is why the SCM was recognized as the primary causal area in Michael's case (and the first muscle I look at in headache patients)[170]. This muscle also has a proprioception function as it helps to balance your head. No muscles controlling your head position would logically cause dizziness.

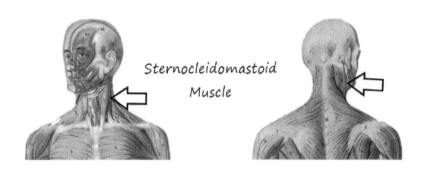

Sternocleidomastoid
Muscle

---

[169] Fancy word for the common cold. Yes, this muscle and how it refers pain onto the sinuses can produce the same nasal symptoms of a common head cold.

[170] Motor dysfunction refers to movement problems as in how the muscle activates or develops weakness. I ask patients if they feel as if they have lost power in a certain muscle. Weakness is not always obvious. Sometimes we find out about weakness in asking patients if they have problems holding a kettle, abnormally dropping their pen or abnormal tiredness in the legs after walking up a staircase.

Trapezius

The next muscle worth a special mention is the trapezius. It gets its name from its shape, a trapezoid. It is a large flat muscle that covers your entire upper back and that has its attachment into the base of your head. You can picture this muscle working like stirrups attached to a horse; the second your head moves forward or tilts downwards, this is the muscle that activates to hold it back. Imagine being the trapezius muscle and your job is holding up the head for the whole day. You would also get tired.

Tired muscles fatigue. Fatiguing muscles develop trigger points. Trigger points refer pain.

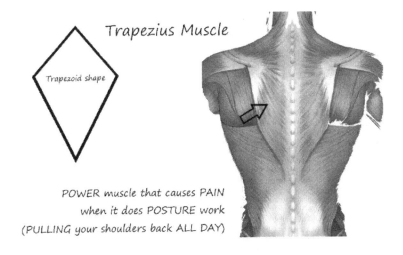

Trapezius Muscle

Trapezoid shape

POWER muscle that causes PAIN
when it does POSTURE work
(PULLING your shoulders back ALL DAY)

The Posterior Cervicals

We now move on to the deeper muscles[171]. You will need a picture like the one below to see where these are, but if I pushed the tip of my finger into the base of your head, it could cover all of them. By applying pressure at different angles, one can try to isolate which is which. The key word here is *try*. This is a painful experience[172].

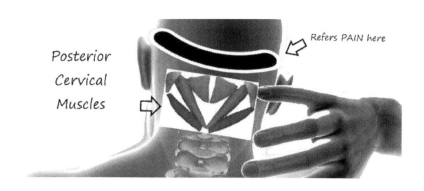

Posterior Cervical Muscles

Refers PAIN here

---

[171] If you care about the specifics, the names of the three suboccipital muscles are the rectus capitis posterior minor, rectus capitis posterior major, and obliquus capitis inferior muscles.

[172] Insert an evil grin here. Patients often ask me if I enjoy inflicting pain on them. *No comment.* Seriously though, the only pleasure that I do get out of it is knowing that the pain is temporary and that it is the start of their recovery.

Ligaments

Ligaments, indirectly, can cause headaches, especially if they have started to limit movement. This is common in the over 40 age group.

The main ligaments you need to know about which are related to the headache realm, are the capsular ligaments. Capsular ligaments are what support every joint in the body by attaching across a joint[173]. These ligaments can become lax or loose due to any traumatic injury, such as heading a soccer ball for instance which, if you watch it in slow motion, causes excessive movement of the neck.

Once a joint has become unstable, the body is going to try support it. It does this by creating muscle tension to support the now loose ligaments. This, over time, results in the joint instability, which causes the body over years to want to fuse the joint as a last-ditch effort to support it. We can see evidence of this on X-rays. This is one of the cycles that we can alter in the long term with Neural Re-Education.

---

[173] Ligaments join bone to bone. Tendons join muscle to bone. An easy way to remember is think of Achilles. In Greek mythology, Achilles was a hero of the Trojan War. He was killed near the end by being shot in the heel by an arrow. Later legends state that Achilles was invulnerable in all his body except for his heel because, when his mother dipped him in the river Styx as an infant, she held him by one of his heels. That is where the injury Achilles' heel comes from, as well as the actual name Achilles tendon.

Membranes

A quick lesson in biomechanics. You have seven neck vertebrae, all of which should help you turn your head to look over your shoulder. However, instead of all seven joints taking equal share of the rotation, most of the rotation happens between the skull and the first vertebrae[174]. This is the same area where the vertebral artery runs (one of the arteries that supplies blood to your brain).

Now if the membrane here begins to calcify as the ligaments above did, the symptoms can be summarized by a cluster of symptoms described in Bow Hunter's Syndrome, where the vertebral arteries in the neck can be compressed by the vertebrae, or other structures. Most often, the C1-2 joint is the most common site. Dizziness, vertigo, headaches, nausea, vomiting, visual disturbances, and imbalance are the most common symptoms.

This is similar to migraines, right? Almost identical. Why have you never heard about this condition? Perhaps because there are not billions to be made from it. From my observations there are currently no over the counter or prescription medications that are indicated.

---

[174] When Bruce Lee breaks people's necks on TV, it is because he can generate enough force to over-rotate that joint. We spoke about this earlier but if I did break your neck with my finger, it would be due to a pathological fracture and the odds are you have cancer." This helps patients relax most of the time.

Joints

Joints have the ability to directly cause headaches, by virtue of their direct link to muscles and the nerves which pass adjacent to them.

I have noticed an influx of patients recently who want to be "cracked" after seeing videos of adjustments on *YouTube*. I am not complaining. I do not mind how people walk through my door; all I care about is that they leave the better for it.

There are two things to understand regarding neck joints.

ONE. The mechanics of a locked joint. We need to get the joint moving. It may take weeks or months to restore normal movement or at least optimal movement. The neuromuscular and mechanical re-education is a timely process that needs to be made informative and patient-centered.

This is because; TWO. A restricted joint will be prone to inflammation and this can irritate the nerves that exit next to the joint.

Nerves

When we speak about the joints, we are interested in the spinal nerves exiting next to the joint. Any irritation to a nerve, for example inflammation in the joint that sits literally next to the nerve, can cause nerve symptoms somewhere else.

I am sure you may have heard about *Sciatica*. Sciatica is pressure on the sciatic nerve in the deep gluteal muscles in the bum. The piriformis muscle can compress the sciatic nerve, referring nerve pain into the leg. The same thing can happen in the head. Compression on or around the occipital nerves can refer pain in the areas where those branches go. Nerve pain can be numbness, tingling, burning, shooting, electric, etc.

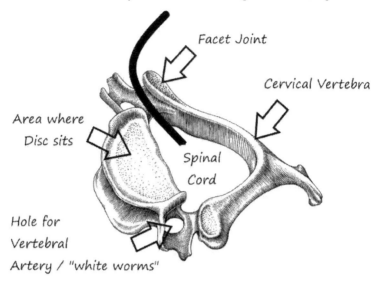

Spinal Nerve, exiting next to the joint

Facet Joint

Cervical Vertebra

Area where
Disc sits

Spinal
Cord

Hole for
Vertebral
Artery / "white worms"

Like sciatica, trigger points in the same muscles through which the nerve exits can cause a remarkably similar *pattern* of pain, but the *characteristics* of the pain are vastly different[175].

---

[175] Diagnostics 101. Ask the right questions. If there is a dull ache, think muscle referred pain. If there is numbness, tingling, burning, electric shocks or shooting pain, think nerve irritation.

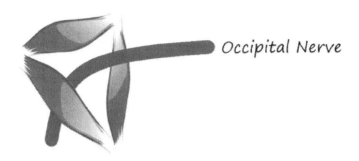

Posterior Cervical Muscles

Occipital Nerve

Posterior Ponticle

Literally meaning *little posterior bridge*, a posterior ponticle is defined as an abnormal small bony bridge which is formed by calcification of the atlantooccipital membrane, (which was mentioned earlier), around the vertebral artery.

Now, on X-rays I have personally taken of headache patients, a large majority have posterior ponticles or partial ponticles, (partial implying that part of the membrane is showing calcification), in a perfect circular pattern. If you use your imagination you can see exactly where the vertebral artery is running.

What it means to me in practice is that the segment has probably been immobile for years, as calcification has developed, among other factors, from lack of movement. *If you do not use it, you lose it.*

I even have a partial ponticle myself, linked to being struck by a car when I was 16 years old. It was probably not rehabilitated properly at the time. I was advised to have rehab, but I thought I knew better, we think we know everything at 16, right?

Why have you never heard about this condition? You are noticing the trend here? Because there are not billions to be made from it; no over the counter or prescription medications are indicated. This is just another observation. (You will have noticed that I copied and pasted that last part from an earlier section.)

Blocked Ears and Sinus Problems

Fairly often patients come in and complain of ear blocking or sinus problems with their headaches. Some patients talk about a clogged or stuffed ear. Allow me to introduce you to the Eustachian tube - the tube that drains your middle ear and sinuses and exits into the back of your throat.

What is so interesting is that I have had numerous patients with this diagnosis or clinical picture, and when upper cervical joint restrictions are corrected, and the muscle tension subsides, they either mostly or completely recover from the symptoms of blocking ears and stuffy sinuses[176].

Most Headaches are Curable

Let us move on before we all develop a headache. The main things I want you to take away from this chapter are:

ONE. Most headaches are treatable, manageable, and largely preventable.

TWO. Headaches cause substantial pain and disability in

---

[176] Blocked ears often have to do with releasing the tension around the Eustachian tubes (where the middle ear drains into the back of your throat). The eustachian tubes help regulate ear pressure and drain excess fluid from the middle ear, moving it to the throat to be eliminated. Remember, wherever pain is referred you can have symptoms, therefore if pain refers over the sinuses, the sinuses stop draining themselves, and sinusitis (stuffy sinus) symptoms present themselves (as seen earlier with the SCM muscle, as one example).

people's daily lives and deliver a high burden and cost to society. The most common headaches diagnosed worldwide are tension-type headache and migraine. However, as I have seen in practice, these terms are often over-diagnosed or improperly diagnosed and patients with pre-existing headaches respond to conservative treatment and respond well. The only conclusion I can come to is that it was not the headache they were originally diagnosed with and in most cases, it came secondarily from the neck.

THREE. If you are not seeing miracles in your treatment within three or four treatments, ask questions, and then obtain a second, third or fourth opinion[177].

FOUR. Practically, it is so important to literally have hands on your patient during their exam. When I have my hands on the base of my patient's head, and exert fingertip pressure into this area, I can often reproduce the symptoms. If your doctor has not touched you during your examination, you are not seeing a doctor, you are seeing a businessman.

Math.

---

[177] Miracles or drastic improvements. I always mention that all we look for is a hint of improvement. Any hint or *window of relief* will mean that we are on the right projection to solving the algorithm.

Point to ponder: If you can reproduce it, you can fix it.

16 : Little *Soix*

Jon's neurological examination findings: Loss
of sensation dermatomal, two-point
discrimination and vibration L4 and L5 on the
right. Absent reflex L4 and L5 right. Grade 4
weakness ankle plantarflexion right. Cranial
nerves NAD. *Something is unquestionably
hitting a nerve.*

The purpose of this chapter is to show a link between
genetics, movement and our health. To do this, let
me share one of the biggest inspirations in my life
and the person who is my constant reminder to always be
humble.

This stage of learning is called: Humility.

May 2016

An 11-month old male infant presents to the Red Cross Children's hospital in Cape Town, South Africa. The patient has symptoms of auditory neuropathy. Hearing tests confirm deafness. The patient has a stridor, muscle weakness is suspected, and respiratory compromise has manifested as diaphragm weakness and vocal cord paralysis. He will require long-term respiratory support via a ventilator, a gastrostomy tube to support feeding. Eventually he will require a PEG[178], and bilateral cochlear implants. With high-dose riboflavin supplementation, he may have limited recovery of motor function. His respiratory chain enzyme studies are abnormal, suggestive of mitochondrial dysfunction.

The above case is my nephew Cameron. Also known as Cammy or Little Soix[179].

He was born with an extremely rare genetic disease called Brown-Vialetto-van Laere syndrome, the first case in Sub-Saharan Africa. It is an *autosomal recessive condition*. Both parents need to have this gene mutation for it to be passed on. That adds to the rareness of the disease, as the chances of both parents having this gene is somewhere in the billionth percentile.

---

[178] Percutaneous Endoscopic Gastrostomy. This is a tube that is passed into a patient's stomach, through the abdominal wall, most commonly to provide a means of feeding when intake through the mouth is not adequate, or possible. It would be nearly impossible for an infant to orally take his maximum dose of vitamin B2 every four hours. This way it can be done while he is asleep. So, as Kaylem would say, you just *squish* the syringe's contents of Riboflavin into his stomach.

[179] Soix (pronounced *soy-ks*) is a nickname. My brother Kaylem, Nicole and I all call each other Soix. Naturally then, Cammy is Little Soix. It was a nickname of mine developed in high school. It started as Mfoif (or Foif for short), which was my isiXhosa nickname. Foif meant "five-head". You see, some would say I have a rather large forehead, which is why my isiXhosa friends at school called me Mfoif as they regarded my forehead ("four-head") as a "five-head". When we saw someone with an even larger forehead than my own, the name Msoix (six-head) was born.

Little Soix's body has altered genes for the way his body transports vitamin B2, which is essential for nerve growth. It mostly affects his brainstem, which is the most important part of the brain. It controls breathing, hearing, swallowing, amongst other important functions for life.

If you were ever blessed enough to meet him, you would find that he is a bright and happy soul. He is an adventurer who loves the water, but should he fall face first into it, he could drown in a mere two inches. He lives with a tracheotomy, which is a permanent hole in his throat so that a ventilator can be attached at night. He has a peg which is a permanent food tube directly into his stomach and he has two artificial cochlear implants so that he can hear.

In 2020, my brother and Nicole had their second boy, Scott, who has already been confirmed to have the same genetic mutation. There was a one in four chance of that happening after the one in billions chance of them both even having the gene.

Take genetics out of it and to me this is proof that your environment affects how cells replicate.

If you think about it, without Little Soix's maximum vitamin dose every four hours, the reality is that he would eventually die. Nerve cells require a certain internal environment to repair and regenerate[180], and without vitamin B2 the internal healing environment is inadequate for that.

We also require an external healing environment to promote cell replication. In Cammy's case, these are the physical and artificial supports of his cochlear implants, PEG and tracheotomy. For patients who are in comas, the physical

---

[180] The same is true for muscles, joints, organs, everything really. If you create the right environment, you will always be healing and repairing to your individual optimum. It really is that simple. And you will see other ways of optimizing these environments in the upcoming chapters.

breathing machine needed to move air in and out of the body, creating a healing environment, is an extreme example of why movement is medicine.

For you and me, it may be different. Our physical exercise could be the means to lowering our stress or inflammation levels, which are the common major causes of toxic internal environments that prevent cell replication (healing). Exercise could merely be there to induce autophagy, which, if you remember, is the body's way of cleaning out damaged cells, that further creates a healing environment to regenerate newer, healthier cells.

Predestination

Our genes are not always our fate. To add to this, let me suggest that being active and eating clean were built into our deepest genetics from the beginning of creation and these things help to make us human. Humans are driven by reason and logic. We can engage in intellectual activities and we have the freedom of choice to change our health habits. We have the conscious ability to make free choices to eat better or to be more active once we know the benefits of them.

For early man there plainly was no option to eat unhealthily before processed food and artificial preservatives were invented. And if our ancestors were lazy, they would have likely died. Those are the genes that have passed on to us.

Sometimes people recognise inherited genes to be a certain reality they must accept, and they live their lives unaware of their ability to change their path. Others have simply become conditioned to poor lifestyle choices that they have inherited from their surroundings. Culturally, we have all been exposed to ways of moving, of eating, and of living, that we carry into our adulthood, and are likely to pass on to our children. That is often why we develop the same diseases as our parents and grandparents, but this does not have to be inevitable.

Even if you have a genetic risk for a disease or a condition, that does not mean you are destined to suffer it. What determines whether it manifests or not are things that are in your control. These include the movement factor, the environmental factor, the diet factor.

We can change our genes if we make changes to our lifestyles. These changes can be powerful and dynamic, and you do not have to wait exceedingly long to see the benefits either. Introducing exercise for instance, has shown to have a positive effect on genetic expressions. To my understanding, if the body's cells are constantly regenerating, you want the environment for replication to be such that it promotes identical replication or better, and exercise helps create this environment.

Here are a few examples. Your skin receives more blood flow when you change to an active lifestyle, so you age less quickly. Your skin does not wrinkle as much. Your heart receives more blood, and you can reverse heart disease. You can decrease your risk of cancers by avoiding the aggravators. Even your sexual organs receive more blood flow, so you increase sexual potency.

Cancer is the ultimate example of how the environment you create within your body effects cell replication. The word 'cancer', from Latin, meaning "crab or creeping ulcer" may be the best description yet, as that is how it spreads. As deadly as cancer is, it is simple to understand. One cell becomes damaged and replicates differently. These become two damaged cells. They replicate to make four. Then eight. Sixteen. You get the idea.

Movement, your diet, and the environment within your body that these create, can prevent damage to cells or prevent the start of them at the very least. The reverse here also applies. When healing happens, we want perfect replication or better replication. Yes, your cells can repair better than before, depending on the environment of healing.

Optimal Healing Environment

In 2018 I contracted Hepatitis A, I suspect, while surfing in Durban. Basically, this means that I probably ingested someone's faeces in some form. What a delicious thought.

Hepatitis is a viral disease that attacks your liver. Hepatitis B and C are the deadly ones with long term complications but contracting Hepatitis A often results in a full recovery. I was the textbook hepatitis picture. I woke up one morning, went to the toilet, and passed what can only be described as flat Coca Cola out of my urethra[181]. Strange.

I then drank coffee, to start my normal morning routine, where going to the toilet is the next step. I then noticed the second mystery of the morning - pale stools. As white as snow. Again, strange. By now I realised something was not right with my liver. The trifactor came when I looked in the mirror and saw that I was a glowing yellow, a real-life character from The Simpsons. I called my doctor, who you will meet in the chapter *The F-word*, and he said he would meet me at the hospital, so I cancelled my appointments for the morning and drove myself over there.

I felt deathly ill. My brother, who had extensive exposure to hepatitis in the government hospital sectors, says that he had never seen hepatic blood levels as high as mine and he does not know how my liver did not fail. Hepatitis is extremely contagious, and I was booked off work for three weeks. It was during this time that I learnt the purpose of being booked off work - which is to rest - and the purpose of avoiding anything that would stress my body - which is to create a healing environment.

---

[181] Here is how you remember it. Your ureter passes from your kidneys *to* your bladder. Your urethra passes *through* your penis.

It was my brother who gave me a stern reminder that my liver is a large organ, and it needs to heal. Rest does not necessarily mean exclusive bed rest; it also means no stressing. In conjunction with that, I followed a liver-friendly diet, which basically means eating anything that the liver does not need to break down too much. Therefore alcohol, sugar, bad carbs, bad fats, dairy, to name a few, were removed from my diet during this time.

The point of this story is that once my immune system had fought the virus off, my body and my liver must have regenerated. What I have noticed now is that I do not feel the effects of alcohol as severely as before. I even joked that I recommend everyone gets hepatitis so that they can also have a regenerated liver. I often had to reiterate the *joking* part.

Exercise and Genes

What is the link between genetics and movement? It is something called the brain-derived neurotrophic factor, or BDNF. When we exercise, the body produces BDNF, which is a natural protein found mainly in the brain. BDNF nourishes nerves in a way. It promotes making new nerves (neurogenesis), protecting nerves (neuroprotection) and regenerating damaged nerve cells (neuroregeneration). In one study, BDNF was literally poured onto a petri dish of neurons, and nerves instantly started sprouting new nerve endings. Adding more exercise would increase hormones responsible for brain plasticity, which would influence your future genetics.

My understanding of exercise and our genetics is that exercise is a part of our genes. We had to adapt to chasing our food and hunting, or physically moving to better climates, or to physically performing manual planting and harvesting of plants.

Essentially, you moved, or you died. And I hear and agree

with the people who say things like *well computers are the future, so our postures will adapt to that*, however we must also consider that it took 2000 years to alter our genes. They are unlikely to evolve dramatically in the 30 years of the financial and transportation revolutions.

Intermittent Fasting

The following chapter is on diet and how I have seen the healing power of clean eating. Besides the actual food you eat, the pattern of your eating is also of importance. Are you a breakfast, lunch and dinner person? Or a six small meals kind of guy or gal? Something that I practice most days is intermittent fasting[182].

Intermittent fasting is an eating pattern where you cycle between periods of eating and fasting. There are many different types of intermittent fasting, the one I utilise most is 16/8. This means that I eat for eight hours, and fast for sixteen. So, I eat dinner at 20:00, and my first meal the next day is at midday.

One of the benefits of exercise, as we saw earlier, is autophagy, (the body removing the bad or damaged cells on its own). You can also train your body to do this with fasting. There are many benefits to this pattern of eating, and I recommend you try it. It may not be for you, but some of the benefits worth mentioning in this chapter are the effect on your genetic makeup.

When you do not eat for a while, your body begins to heal its own cells, makes changes to some hormone levels, and

---

[182] It is not only important what you eat, but how (and when) you eat it – the frequency and amounts of food consumed. For instance, in South Africa we have huge meal portions. I remember my first fine dining experience, I thought that we had three starters. This is a reminder we should eat to nourish ourselves, not to merely be full.

replicates your cells better and more effectively. It is as simple as that.

Blood levels of insulin drop, which facilitates fat burning. One of the side benefits is weight loss. The blood levels of human growth hormone may increase as much as five-fold. Higher levels of this hormone accelerate fat burning and muscle gain, and they also have numerous other benefits in healing the body. (Remember from earlier – there are similar changes when you sleep more.)

The most interesting finding is the potential changes to your general gene expression. In other words, how your genes will show themselves as physical or physiological traits. Autophagy is the means through which the body can remove damaged cells and recycle parts of them toward cellular repair and cleaning. The better your body does this, the better longevity and protection against disease you will have.

To wrap up this chapter in a nutshell, *we can change the expression of our genes*. We can change what cells look like after they have replicated. We can alter tumour-suppressing genes and tumour-activating genes by what we put into our bodies, and by what we do with our bodies in the form of movement and eating clean.

So, even if you have been dealt a bad genetic hand, you can still reshuffle it somewhat with a few changes. If this were a betting game, it would be time to go all in.

Point to ponder: Have you always been
nervous to make a change because you thought
that nothing could be done?

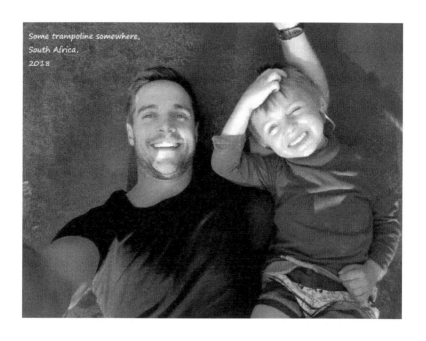

Some trampoline somewhere,
South Africa,
2018

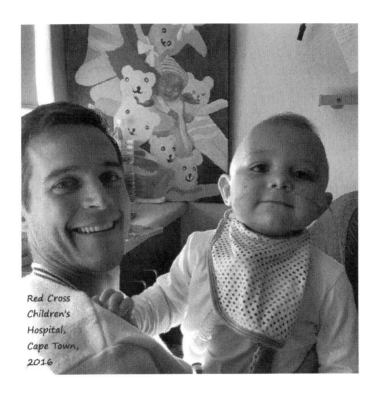

Red Cross
Children's
Hospital,
Cape Town,
2016

17 : Eat Clean

Jon's primary diagnosis: L4/5 disc prolapse
posterolateral on the right. Begin conservative
management and NRE protocol a.s.a.p. under
close monitoring. If no response, refer. *He
should respond well; most disc patients do not
need operations.*

O ne of the most powerful tools to combat
inflammation and stress does not come from the
pharmacy, but from the earth. The main objective
of clean eating is to decrease inflammation and not to add
stress to an already stressed internal environment.

Before we even begin, remember that there is no *one* or
correct diet for anyone. The same is true with exercise
programs, rehabilitation plans and recovery methods, as we
have already seen in this book. Everyone is wired uniquely,
and everyone will respond differently to different stimuli. I can
merely offer what has worked for me, and more importantly,
clinically, I can offer you what has worked for hundreds of my
patients who have followed the same guidelines.

About three years ago I started to take my diet seriously. Not that it was horrendous, but I had a few bad habits, so I decided to practice what I preach and eat clean. A side motivator was that I have always been concerned about cancer because both my grandparents on my father's side died of cancer[183]. I wondered if things would have been different had they known the link between diet and this dreadful disease.

We have all seen domestic cats and dogs with growths and tumours on them. Have you ever wondered why this happens? I believe it is because only household animals eat human made food.

We come from a conservational hunting family and as the youngest in the family I have had to skin many wild animals after they have been shot. One thing that we have never seen on wild animals is a growth or tumour, inside or on the body. We see abscesses of course, from injuries or puncture wounds, and obviously wild animals cannot take antibiotics, but we are yet to see a cancerous tumour[184]. The association between human-made food and cancer is incontestable.

---

[183] Many things from my family have personally inspired me to eat better. My grandfather died from colon cancer. So did 16 of his brothers. This is one of my reasons for avoiding foods that sit in your gut, things like processed foods and refined carbs. My dad suffers from kidney stones, so I avoid sugar and make sure my water intake is sufficient. You do not need personal family stories to motivate your choice to eat clean. You could simply steal mine or use other examples in this chapter.

[184] It makes me feel better to add the word conservational to hunting. For the vegans reading this book, let me explain a few things. In South Africa, most of the farms have no lions or other predators to keep the number of antelope under control. Antelope breed extremely efficiently. They also eat massive amounts of grass. The reality is that if you do not hunt, the number of antelope become too many for the amount of grass available to feed on. The math is such that if you do not hunt, the whole ecosystem will suffer as animals begin to die from starvation.

My cousin Don had cancer. Hairy Cell Leukaemia. We raced a few adventure races together, and he has represented South Africa at the world championships level before. Adventure races use navigation and checkpoints to ultimately cover hundreds of kilometres over multiple days of racing. These races include running, paddling, and cycling, to name a few. Don has been described as a diesel engine, and I have witnessed him display his stamina and endurance. So, when he was diagnosed with cancer, he focused on overcoming this challenge just the same. After the initial chemotherapy had decreased the blood markers in his body, he opted to halt the growth of the cancer naturally. He had a diet consisting of only homemade green juices; spinach, celery, cucumber, apple, kiwi, ginger etc. All refined carbohydrates were exchanged for vegetable options, and no artificial sugar was permitted, only honey if needed. Ten years later he is still in remission. The lesson here is that it is possible to starve the cancer, so it cannot grow. Similarly, if you starve inflammation, it cannot grow. In obtaining his permission to write about him, he reminded me of the life-altering magnitude of clean eating. He also reminded me about the essentiality of a family support system, finding joy and the active choice of wanting to heal - more on these later.

If you starve cancer, it cannot grow. If you starve inflammation, it cannot spread.

We now know that our bodies are always regenerating. Every cell, every tissue and every organ is regenerating, and the quality of the regeneration is partly reliant on your diet. Your diet will change the landscape of your internal healing environment. You are *literally* what you eat.

If you put poison into your body, you will get sick.

As with any subject on social media, everyone has much to say. When you bring up the subject of diets with people however, they either have strong opinions and judgments on the subject or they keep noticeably quiet. Instagram models like to think of themselves as scientists. While veganism or

301

plant-based diets seem to embrace sugar, sweeteners and additives, as long as they are not derived from animals. I believe you should research your own dietary experience, absorb what is useful, reject what is useless and add what is specifically your own and what adds to your health.

I have become meticulous about my diet. My family constantly tell me to *live a little* and eat everything in moderation. The scientist in me knows all the reasons to eat clean and the long-term benefits of doing so, so how could I not?

It is worthwhile mentioning here that you will not see the benefits of any healthy habit immediately. You may see weight loss as a relatively short-term benefit. (The world around us, television and media marketing, have made us subconsciously desire *quick fixes* for almost everything.) What I have witnessed in my own life and in private practice, is that there is no substitute for being consistent, and being patient. Your healthy internal environment will take years to fully mature - like a good wine. The moral of this short story is start as soon as you can, make one small change at a time, and be patiently consistent.

That said, I am all for the odd cheat day where no rules apply, like when I am a guest at someone's house. Showing gratitude and embracing what my hosts are offering me are more important to me than being a stuck-up, know-it-all at a dinner party.

Apart from movement, one of the most essential things I can advise someone is to eat clean. I have mentioned before that I am not a dietitian and therefore, I cannot give you an eating plan. The reality is that there is no one diet to which everybody will respond. But I can tell you how I eat, and how it has changed my entire life. Every aspect of my life has been improved by backing a clean eating lifestyle - coupled with exercise of course. I feel better, look better, perform better athletically and vocationally, sleep better, have more energy, and focus better. Everything in my life really is better than what it was before I cleaned up my diet. Making some changes to your diet may be the most prosperous financial investment you can make for your body, and well worth the effort.

Professor Tim Noakes has always had my utmost respect and admiration because he breaks bad science. He turns heads and takes no prisoners in his bold approach to educating the public. He also argues that there is not one study that proves any diet conclusively right or wrong, since it is impossible to undertake such a study. To perform that kind of study you would have to lock around fifty thousand people up in a hospital jail for around forty years. This would be difficult and costly, if not ethically suspect and physically challenging. Rather, you must look at the totality of the medical evidence. In doing this, Professor Noakes made a 180° about-face from campaigning for high carbohydrate diets to low carbohydrate ones.

The *low carb guru* as he is known to some, was taken to task by the Health Professionals Council of South Africa for giving "unconventional" low carb advice to a breastfeeding mother on Twitter. After examining the science in depth, Professor Noakes knew that what he suggested was accurate, and the court ruled as such.

The mind knows not what the tongue wants. We have all been there. We have a sugary binge eating weekend, and a few days later we wake up with stiff joints or, worse if you are young, a pimple. The food we ate days before has worked its way through our systems and has become integrated with new cells as they are duplicating. In joints, this may lead to inflammatory responses. In the skin, it may lead to mucus build-up as the body tries to expel the toxins, also known as pimples.

To me, clean eating, like movement, is defined as doing what you were designed to do. We are designed to eat what we can grow, find, or, if we are skilful enough, what we can hunt. And in the freshest way possible. Recently I have added to that phrase and it can now be summarized to *eat as if you did not own a fridge.* No fridge means eat things as fresh as possible - what can be grown seasonally. This means fewer artificial preservatives, less 21st century dairy, and eating more things that can go off easily. It means eating meat less frequently. What I have noticed is how this diet supports an anti-inflammatory type of diet, limiting food that prolongs acute inflammation, sustains chronic inflammation or can, in itself, cause inflammation.

During my preparation for the New York marathon, I followed the guidelines in this chapter almost perfectly. In real life, I find following these rules 90% of the time is more than beneficial for my health. In addition, I consumed no alcohol for the five weeks leading up to the race.

Nutrition advisors try to build a perfect diet around an imperfect world. There is no way we should be able to eat everything, all year around. It is just not natural. It really is that simple. Look at humans 2000 years ago. They would eat off the fat of the land, and often go for hours or days without eating. It is interesting that 'intermittent fasting' is considered a 'new' dietary approach when it is simply how our ancestors ate.

Here is a patient example.

October 2016

Tyrion Lannister, a 45-year-old male patient presents to the clinic. Vertically challenged guy with a disturbing family history resulting in many psychological traumas.

Tyrion presents with generalised pain and a previously diagnosed chronic pain syndrome and Rheumatoid arthritis[185]. He has been prescribed antidepressant medication as well as benzodiazepines (anxiety medication). He is reluctant to do any exercise for fear of flaring up the pain. He describes a diet predominantly high in refined carbohydrates, sugar, preservatives and alcohol.

We first rule out Chiari malformations and spina bifida (both effect the spinal cord).

Fast forward three months. Tyrion responded to a NRE protocol. He has definitive windows of relief. Pain is less frequent and less severe. He is off antidepressant medication. Tyrion still uses benzodiazepines. Patient's ADL have drastically improved[186]. He has made no changes to his diet. Tyrion has successfully started considerably basic Zone 2 exercise, core activation exercises and stretching.

Fast forward another three months. Tyrion comes for treatment every second week now. Patient continuing with exercise and ADL improving. Patient's pain is now two out of ten, previously and consistently at six out of ten, and pain is less frequent. Patient has reduced refined carbohydrates and alcohol quantities. Stricter dietary changes are advised.

Fast forward another three months. Tyrion following an anti-inflammatory diet. Treatment frequency every four weeks now. Tyrion is off medication completely. Pain at one out of ten when experienced and relievable at home with stretching, exercise and using heat packs.

---

[185] Abbreviated as RA. When a patient presents with this or if you suspect this, you never adjust the patient's neck. It is a strange disease with a broad array of symptoms. One of the things that happens in RA is the transverse ligament of the second vertebrae becomes weak. In other words, adjusting the patient at that level would be reckless. That said, as with other chronic pain syndromes such as fibromyalgia, osteoarthritis, Lupus and irritable bowel syndrome, pain relief can be achieved by applying the gate control mechanism of manual treatment. Pain relief can also be achieved using diet, particularly an *anti-inflammatory diet*.

[186] ADL, activity of daily living. This is what we focus on. If a patient can perform daily tasks easier, more efficiently, with less pain and perform tasks that were previously impossible, that is significant. This means we are on the right track.

The good-to-knows:

ONE. This was the case that opened my eyes to the real power of clean eating.

TWO. The diet change was the primary healing agent that tilted the seesaw in our favour in this case. As soon as the patient changed his diet, we observed a significant improvement in treatment outcomes.

My Diet Summarized

Mostly plant based (*If you can grow it or find it, you can eat it*).

There are no artificial sugars (*These are simply poison*).

There is no white flour or processed foods *(You process all the goodness out of the food)*.

There are no artificial preservatives *(Limit food that has a shelf life)*.

Fish and free-range meat only *(AND, only as frequently as if I were catching or hunting them myself. That is how our ancestors did it)*.

Keep it simple.

My aim is to follow these guidelines for myself 90% of the time. I have found there is so much merit in also having the bad things every now and again. Why? It reminds my body what bad is, and it maintains my body's resistance to those things.

ADD	LIMIT
Fruit	Sugar
Vegetable	Refined carbohydrates
Nuts, seeds	Artificial preservatives
Water	Mass produced dairy
Fish and free-range meats	Meat from animals that have been fed human-made foods
If you could grow it yourself or find it in nature	

Start shopping at health food stores, buy organic, and be diligent about reading labels to identify 'hidden' ingredients, with names that fool you into thinking you are buying something healthy.

I have consulted many dietitians on this. My summary of what they say regarding fruit would be a maximum of two portions of fruit a day, where one portion is roughly one medium fruit or half a cup. Also, it is important to rotate / vary the types of fruit and vegetables you eat, as no one fruit contains all the nutrients you need.

Meat and other animal products produce inflammation in the body. Most plant foods are anti-inflammatory in nature and therefore lead to a quicker recovery time after exercise and injury.

Joint pain, bloating and foggy thoughts are not imagined symptoms, they are often the result of improper diet. Make eliminations. Start with wheat, then dairy, then sugar. These are the most inflammatory foods.

Anti-Inflammatory Diet

One major part of your recovery-driven lifestyle needs to be clean eating, the physical act of what you put inside yourself. The following are guidelines that I have personally followed, based on advice, reading, researching and courses I have attended. A practical way to begin eating clean would be to try removing or adding something from your diet for around three weeks to see how your body responds. Body adaption to change does not happen overnight. Also, you will most likely experience some sort of withdrawal symptoms, such as headaches and general digestion changes from your norm[187].

Sugar

The main foodstuff I am against, and the first thing I pay close attention to in my diet, is sugar. Sugar is probably worse for you than cocaine. Only once I cut sugar largely out of my diet did I notice what was always there. The classic teaching is that you do not know what you have until it has gone. The opposite is true with sugar. *You know what you have when it has gone.*

My eyes were opened when I heard of a medical procedure from a patient of mine who had been diagnosed with thyroid cancer. There is a blood test that can show whether you have thyroid cancer or not; however, the scan of your thyroid may come back and show no abnormalities. In this instance, the Positron Emission Tomography (PET) scan is a way to create pictures of organs and tissues inside the body. A small amount of a radioactive sugar substance is injected into the patient's body. This sugar substance is taken up by the cells that use the most energy. Cancer cells tend to use energy actively and therefore absorb more of the radioactive substance. A scanner then detects this substance and produces images of the inside of the body. Basically, your thyroid lights up like a Christmas tree on this scan after you have had the sugar. It demonstrated so clearly to me that cancer cells feed on sugar. After this

---

[187] Frequency and texture of your number two's during toilet time. Awkward.

realisation, I decided to cut added sugar out of my life almost completely.

Eating too much sugar is bad for your health. How is that for scientific terminology? It has been linked to an increased risk of many diseases, including obesity, heart disease, type 2 diabetes and cancer. One of the reasons is because many foods contain hidden sugars, including some foods that you would not even consider to be sweet. Marketing does not help either, often the "light" or "low-fat" products contain more sugar than the regular versions.

Most people compare fructose with its friend glucose. But they are not friends at all. Glucose is so critical for life that our livers can produce it when it is in short supply. It is the same as cannabinoids and endorphins - your body has receptors only for substances that it can make on its own.

If you are still not convinced about cutting out sugar, think of it as the same as alcohol. Replace the word sugar in your brain with alcohol. I assume you would not add alcohol to your cereal. You also would not instinctively give alcohol to a child. Although sugar does not display the same short-term toxic effects as alcohol, it reiterates all the same long-term toxic effects on our health. If ever there was a time for a complete societal shift away from sugar consumption, it is now.

When we eat sugar, our blood glucose levels temporarily rise. This is great for an acute episode of body function, but when that level drops, your body goes into a mini shock. Your body begins to hunger. The natural survival technique would be finding more sugar. And so, the cycle continues.

Sugar occurs naturally in all foods that contain carbohydrates, such as fruits, vegetables, and grains. Consuming whole foods that contain natural sugar is completely fine. That should not be disputed. Plant foods also have high amounts of fibre, essential minerals, and antioxidants, and other green leafy vegetables contain calcium too. Since your body digests these foods slowly, the sugar in them offers a steady supply of energy to your cells and you limit the spikes in your blood glucose levels just described. The real problem occurs when you consume too much added sugar; the sugar that food manufacturers add to products to increase flavor or extend shelf life.

Bad Carbs

The next alteration I made to my diet was to restrict bad carbs - refined carbohydrates. Bad carbs include sugars and refined grains that have been stripped of all bran, fibre, and nutrients (all the good stuff). These include white bread, pizza dough, pasta, pastries, white flour, white rice, sweet desserts, and many breakfast cereals. There are numerous reasons for this, but you do not need to look too far as nature often tells us everything you need to know.

Regarding carb intake in general. I try limit mine. I find this helps me stay lean. The extreme forms of low carb diets are the *Atkins*, *Ketogenic* and *Banting* diets. I know many patients and friends who use these diets, and if it works for them, I recommend continuing.

My friend Roche is a farmer in the Eastern Cape of South Africa, and he told me something profound - yet which is common sense. If he wants to fatten up his sheep on the farm, he feeds them carbs. If he wants them to lose weight, he gets the sheepdogs to chase them and make them walk up and down the mountain. I shall leave it at that. As a sports person, staying lean is always important to me, but from a health aspect, the bad carbs are often hidden with added sugar too.

Alcohol

There is research that says one glass of wine a day prevents cancer and other research which says that one glass of wine a day causes cancer. When this happens, we need to break bad science again.

There is no questioning that alcohol is not good for your body. It is a toxin and therefore your body will *stress* to break it down. From what I have read, sugar is worse for your body long-term, so pick your poison so to say. This may sound controversial now, but if that glass of red wine helps you relax and be less anxious, or helps you be more social, those far outweigh the negative effects.

Water

Drink it.

How much should you drink is the question. Two litres a day, I find, is a happy medium. Professor Tim Noakes' research on water intake suggests you should drink when you are thirsty. That is the natural survival advice. Simply drinking water when you feel like it is all you need to perform at your best personal capacity.

When starting a NRE protocol with a patient, I always recommend drinking more water than they usually drink. The main reason for this is that releasing muscle trigger points and moving immobile joints will release metabolites into the blood stream. Your kidneys filter the metabolites in the bloodstream using water.

Meat

All protein originally comes from plants. The cow you eat, ate only plant products, and the protein stored in its muscles comes from plants. Why not just cut out the middleman? Before I get judged, let me say that I do eat red meat. Probably once a week. Majority of my meat intake is fish.

The bottom line is that there are some nutrients that you cannot get from plants alone. Therefore the veganism and vegetarian diets would need to supplement with these. In my head, that is worse for you compared to eating the odd steak, as supplements need to contain preservative agents to keep shelf life, and the nutrient is often not naturally produced. (This logic is how I sleep at night.)

Regarding protein, there is a massive misconception in nutrition that you only obtain protein only from meat products. As far as the quality of protein is concerned, I always thought that animal protein was superior to plant protein. The breakdown products of proteins are amino acids and there are a few essential amino acids that are all found in plant proteins too.

As with any mega money market, if there is money to be made from something, there will be people claiming that it is safe. The news outlets and tabloids will always enthusiastically report any story that suggests people can carry on with habits they enjoy. Worldwide, people are eating more protein than they need, often to the detriment of other nutrients, such as fibre.

I believe that if we are eating meat, it should be fish from the wild or, similarly, animals that roam free and eat off the land only. (Conservational hunting as I mentioned earlier.)

Fibre

To add fibre to your diet, add vegetables, whole-grain products, fruits, and legumes such as beans and peas.

There are two kinds of fibre: insoluble fibre, which is important in the digestive system, and soluble fibre, which is important in our blood streams. Diets high in both kinds of fibre tend to be bulky, and since fibre itself does not contribute calories, foods high in fibre tend to contain fewer calories in the same volume of food. Therefore, eat more volume with less calories.

Fibre seems to be the one dietary component that affords

some protection against nearly every chronic disease known. That makes for good reading.

Dairy

This is always a hot topic to debate. If your only reason to drink dairy is calcium, then I say that there are better forms of calcium out there, that contain less preservatives (the fact is that dairy is a form of calcium). If you love the taste or simply ingest large amounts of milk, then I say practice moderation.

One of the reasons I would give to consume dairy is for gut health. Dairy in its most raw form promotes this, as good bacteria promote a healthy gut. This is where raw yogurt comes in handy. Yogurt is made from milk, with a touch of bacteria to kick off the fermenting process. It contains probiotics, which are live microorganisms like those in your gut. And you will see now how important gut health is to pain management.

In terms of cheese. I love, and I recommend, blue cheese. The blues are not particularly nutrient-dense, but they do offer a good source of protein, calcium, vitamin A and vitamin K2. Vitamin K2, rarely spoken about, has an osteoprotective effect (protects bones) by promoting bone formation[188]. As a chiropractor, therefore, I would recommend these types of cheeses, also for their effect on gut health.

---

[188] Remember that every cell in our body is always replicating. Just think about that for a second. Your bones are constantly making new bone cells (think about how a bunion at the base of your big toe slowly grows bigger or how leg bones can slowly become bow-shaped). This process happens from the inside, where the bone marrow is, and extends outwards to the surface of the bone. Replication, repair, and healing of any cell happens best in an optimal internal healing environment. K2 is one of those vitamins that creates a good environment for bone formation. In my line of work, this is gold. During a NRE protocol, clean eating is essential to aid the process of repair at a cellular level.

Gut Health

An unhealthy gut lining may allow partially digested food, toxins, antigens, or bacteria inside it, to penetrate the tissues around it. From here, these toxins enter the blood stream. This is called a 'leaky gut'. This may trigger inflammation and changes in the normal bacteria that could lead to problems within the digestive tract and even further down the line. Diets that are low in fibre, high in sugar and high in saturated fats, have been identified as initiators of a leaky gut. Heavy alcohol use and stress also seem to disrupt this balance.

The easiest way to treat and prevent this would be to lower stress levels and to combine this with clean eating. But to be leaky-gut specific, avoid foods with active lectins. Lectins are a type of protein. Foods containing active lectins, in their raw state, can cause negative side effects. In nature, lectins defend plants. In human digestion, lectins resist the legume from being broken down in the gut and can damage the inner lining. Ultimately, this can cause leaky-gut and lead to excess inflammation in the body. Eating foods with a high number of active lectins is extremely rare as they are not typically eaten raw.

Why is a leaky gut important? It is one of the largest contributors to chronic pain.

Omega 3

As with a leaky gut, the ratio of Omega 3 to Omega 6 is causally linked to inflammation and is hence another major contributor to chronic pain. We will see this in the next chapter.

Eat Clean

As a Health Coach, I have been intensely aware for a long

time of how many dietary myths and mistaken beliefs persist about what clean eating really is.

When it comes to diet, choose food in its most natural form. Generally speaking, the more it has been processed the more goodness has been taken out of it. Most importantly, eat mindfully, by choosing to balance what you want and enjoy, with a focus on what your body needs first. And from that, (I believe and bear witness to this), you will achieve a physical, emotional and spiritual balance, which is the ultimate state of health.

Start today. Make a change. *You can never get enough of what you do NOT need.*

Below is piece written for this book by holistic nutritionist Natalie Jackson. She is someone from whom I learnt a great deal in perfecting my diet and she has an astounding story herself in curing her autoimmune disease through her diet alone.

I did not realise that health was all I really need until I realised it is all I have.

It is undeniable that 'health' is a fashionable trend, and it has, as a result, become increasingly challenging to decipher which trend to follow. In my pursuit, I came across the concept of "Holistic health" and found what I deem to be the most effective and sustainable choice one could make when it comes to diet. Why? When it comes to prioritizing your health, the most simple and effective way to ensure a positive end result is to assess how much of what you are consuming in your diet positively adds to your health status.

When adopting this lifestyle, you choose to take the wheel of your health when it comes to preparing, ordering or choosing a meal, by asking yourself this one simple question: "What can I add to this meal, to support my body's needs for optimal functioning?" For the answer to this I like to turn to the wisdom of Dr Michael Gregor. In his book, titled "How not to die", he lists the 8 daily essentials to add to your daily meals. They are:

1. Whole grains and starchy vegetables. 2. Beans and other legumes. 3. Berries. 4. Other fruits. 5. Cruciferous vegetables. 6. Leafy greens. 7. Non-starchy vegetables. 8. Nuts and seeds.

All these essentials have been found to have profoundly positive effects on your overall health, as they have the vitamins, minerals and macros needed to support the functioning of all your body's interdependent systems.

Food is medicine, and if every time you eat something, you think of it in that way, I can guarantee you, your relationship with food and with your body image will change entirely.

Point to ponder: If you starve cancer or inflammation, they cannot spread, so what are you adding or taking away from your diet today?

Inflammatory Foods

DECREASES INFLAMMATION	INCREASES INFLAMMATION
OMEGA 3 *Fish such as salmon, mackerel, herring, and sardines Nuts and seeds such as flaxseed, chia seeds, and walnuts*	ACTIVE LECTINS *Raw beans, raw lentils, raw soybeans, raw peanuts, wheat[189]*
VITAMIN D *Fish such as salmon, tuna, and mackerel Fish liver oils*	SUGAR *Soft drinks, sweets, chocolate, some cereals, cakes, doughnuts, pastries, biscuits*
RESVERATROL *Grapes, grape juice, peanuts, cocoa, blueberries, bilberries, and cranberries*	PROCESSED MEATS *Smoked meats, ham, bacon, processed sausage, biltong[190]*

[189] Before you call me out or quote me from earlier "if you could grow it or find it in nature you should add it to your diet", there are some exceptions. Foods containing active lectins can survive human digestion and cause inflammation (explained in detail in the next chapter). Legumes, of course, have many nutritional benefits as seen in the left side of this table and throughout this chapter. Cooking, boiling, or soaking in water for several hours, can inactivate most lectins found in the food. For this reason, as difficult as it is for me to say this, raw peanut butter is not good for you, as it contains active lectins.

[190] This is a South African dried meat, like American jerky.

DECREASES INFLAMMATION	INCREASES INFLAMMATION
HERBS *Curcumin, turmeric, cardamom, cayenne pepper, dill, fresh ginger, parsley, sage, rosemary, oregano, cloves*	EXCESSIVE ALCOHOL
MALIC ACID *Apricots, blackberries, blueberries, cherries, grapes, peaches, pears, plums, citrus*	REFINED CARBOHYDRATES *All processed foods* *Sweets, bread, pasta, pastries, biscuits, cakes, soft drinks*
COENZYME Q10 *Meats, fish, nuts, vegetable oils.*	TRANS FATS *French fries, fried fast foods, margarine, all pastries, cakes, cookies, doughnuts*
A-LIPOIC ACID *Spinach, broccoli, yams, brussels sprouts, carrots and beets.* *Animal liver*	
MAGNESIUM *Green leafy vegetables, such as spinach, legumes, nuts, seeds*	
CARNITINE *Red meat, fish, poultry, and milk*	

18 : Pain

Jon's secondary diagnosis: Left chronic medial
meniscus tear, possible bucket handle. Treat
concomitantly with disc treatment, NRE
protocol and begin rehabilitation as soon as
patient's back is pain-free. If no resolution,
refer for orthopaedic opinion. *Simple
mechanics really.*

In this chapter I discuss natural and holistic ways you
can manage your own pain, from home and for free.
First, we need to understand what pain is and the role it
plays in our bodies. These guidelines are from my personal
and professional experiences. Tried and tested.

Pain can literally be crippling. I have seen grown men cry.
Pain, after all, is the most common reason for people to book
an appointment to see me. And seeking the ecstasy of *pain
relief* is the primary reason people keep coming back. Pain can
also be the most enlightening source of information.

Let me explain. When you are in pain, you often move the
way you should always have moved.

For example, as you hurt your back, the acute pain will bring a muscle spasm to protect it for 72 hours[191], and during this time you will move like a retirement home regular. Something as simple as bending to pick up a coffee cup will force you to bend your knees, push your bum out and possibly use one hand on your knee as a support. But this tells you something; that is that this is the correct way we all should bend. We all too often, and too quickly, bend with our spines and not with our hips and our pelvis. Refer to most of the concepts from earlier that speak about moving the way we were designed to move. If we do not, wear and tear takes place at a faster rate.

The Pain Dilemma

I am grateful for pain because it is the body's mechanism to make us aware that something is not right, and we can seek help to diagnose the problem. However, in all honesty, pain is a rather unhelpful indicator of dysfunction in the body[192].

The first reason for this is that pain is different for every person. I have seen the most radical spinal changes on X-rays where the patient presents with no history of pain. The other side of the coin is where I have seen the mildest spinal changes and the patient is in agony.

Secondly, pain is often the last symptom to present and the first to go away. The analogy is that of the straw that broke the camel's back; every day more straw was added onto the back

---

[191] Acute inflammation normally lasts up to 72 hours. Three days. You are going to be sore for the two days after an injury of any sort. Try not freak out when you experience pain. Buy yourself some time by applying some tips from this chapter, and the acute phase passes quicker than you think.

[192] You have seen this pop up in many chapters in this book. In different forms. In diagnostics, pain is as useful as a pork roast at a vegan convention. Or as useful as Anne Frank's drum kit.

of a camel, and eventually one single piece of straw was the one that broke the camel's back. Now, was it that last piece of straw that did it, or was it the kilograms of straw that were loaded on before that broke the camel's back? It is obviously the prolonged added weight that did it. Similarly, the spine takes wear and tear, over years, and by the time pain is experienced, there is often already years of dysfunction[193].

Now preventing and managing pain is an important aspect of health care, but it is not the only aspect we should pay attention to when listening to our bodies. If you merely seek pain relief, you need simply to take the strongest pain blocker you can find. However, that will do absolutely nothing for you in the long term. Health should not be viewed only as being in a state of no pain. Being pain-free is the by-product of a functional body. True health is having an internal healing environment that can efficiently recover from disease, illness and pain, when they arrive.

Psychological factors play a big role too. In chronic pain disorders, pain is perceived in different anatomic locations such as lower back, head region, abdomen, and chest, I see this regularly.

---

[193] The worst disc injury that I have seen, happened to a patient who bend down to pick up his coffee cup from a coffee table. He needed urgent surgery. The MRI of the lower back showed that the disc contents basically *exploded* into the spinal cord. From simply bending forward, makes no sense, except for the fact he had years of poor posture and no advice on preventive methods. You have education in your hands right now, maybe you could save someone's spine by informing them.

Discomfort vs Pain

Discomfort and pain are different in purpose. Discomfort, for example, is what any runner experiences. Often the first few minutes of running feel as if you are trying to get rusty hinges moving, but this discomfort is often from stiff muscles. It may not indicate dysfunction. Towards the end of a run, discomfort is often the body fatiguing.

I explain to patients when they start exercising again after their injury, that they may need to work through discomfort for a while. The healing muscles and joints will be weaker and will therefore fatigue quicker. This results in discomfort. It is not harmful to do exercise through discomfort, as long as you know *exactly* what pain means or where pain begins. And as long as you stay in Zone 2, of course.

There are a few indicators to look for to ascertain when you are leaving the realm of discomfort and entering the realm of pain. The most important one is that pain will alter your movement pattern. For runners, this may be a limp. For swimmers with shoulder pain, this may be loss of strength and limited reach. For other types of exercise, this may be inability to load the joint properly or stretch the muscle to full length. You get the point.

If you exercise through pain, you will teach the body bad habits rather than restore normal movement, and this will ultimately lead to pain down the line. As far as exercising through discomfort is concerned, it is essential to stay in Zone 2. I need to reiterate this. The only exercise done with discomfort should be low-impact, easy, Zone 2 exercise.

The function of pain is to protect you from hurting yourself even more than you already have. The problem comes when a patient's only goal is to escape the pain. By taking pain killers one tends to forget that there is a problem and the need for the most important part of returning to normal - *Neural Re-Education*.

Teach the brain what normal feels like, again. And again.

Clinically, I find that pain is often the last symptom to

arrive. The changes we see on X-rays, and physical findings during the consultation, take years to present. Pain, on the other hand, normally takes only days or weeks. Where was the pain when the wear and tear started? This is the important thing to remember here. Degeneration of the spine (or any body function) is often disguised as day to day discomfort, symptoms that we all get used to. Things like stiffness, fatigue, mild headaches, or mood changes[194].

Although pain is an easy symptom to treat, the restoration of long-term function and maintaining a healing environment within one's body is what takes discipline and a little bit of toughening up.

Pain is Subjective

The concept of pain has changed from a one-dimensional to a multi-dimensional entity, involving sensory, cognitive, motivational, and affective qualities.

The International Association for the Study of Pain says that pain is "An unpleasant sensory and emotional experience associated with actual or potential tissue damage or described in terms of such damage."

It is also possible for a person to experience 'Allodynia', which is pain from a painless stimulus. An example of this is phantom pain, experienced in a part of the body that has been amputated. Or, as depicted in the film *Kickass,* people can have severe pain insensitivity from abnormalities in the nervous system, such as damage to the nerves. These can include a spinal cord injury, or diabetes.

---

[194] Moodiness, or being abnormally irritable. Feeling like you do not want to do exercise. Laziness. These are some of the symptoms to look out for. Pain does weird things. A loving and caring guy asks his girlfriend: *"When you are feeling moody, would you like space or would you like more of my attention?"* Her answer: *"Yes".*

The description of pain I relate to the most is by McCaffery and Pasero (from 1999), who offered a clinically useful definition: "Pain is whatever the experiencing person says it is."

Once a body part has a perceived pain for an area or joint, my job is to help the patient re-educate the body towards normal movement. With enough patience in the process, we will firstly increase function, and secondly, decrease the emotional reaction to previous pain in that area. The various conscious and unconscious responses to both sensation and perception, including the emotional responses, add further definition to the overall concept of pain.

If you take anything from this chapter take the fact that low back pain and neck pain are often a result of a muscle spasm protecting the area, or from inflammation of the area. More often than not, it is a combination of the two.

I have found that one of the most effective treatment protocols for both muscle spasm and inflammation is physical movement. In my opinion, the best additions to this are heat and ice application, and the best prevention approach is Neural Re-Education.

With the approach of a NRE protocol, I will often explain to patients that we will manage their pain relatively quickly. The pain may however last a short while longer than if the patient had taken strong pain killers, but the pain killer is only numbing the pain and it often comes back soon. At the very least, a NRE protocol will help the future painful episodes. When the same pain comes back, (and it often does), it will be less severe and last nowhere nearly as long as previous episodes. A simple heat pack application, a stretch and good night's sleep will often alleviate the reoccurred pain. An outcome like this, is priceless in my book, both literally and figuratively.

A decrease in pain can be attributed to a decrease in inflammation. A decrease in pain is also attributed to the perception of pain being less because you are experiencing non-painful stimulus again.

The following pain management strategies are what I have found to be most beneficial for the management of my own pain. I have physically experienced effective pain management by adding these to my life[195].

Gate Control Theory

These three words are a basic summary of how I help my patients with pain management. The simplest example of the gate control theory would be bumping your shin on an unclosed dish washer door. The first thing you would naturally do is rub the area. That is instinctive. A specific part of your brain experienced painful stimulus from the bump, and immediately afterwards the rubbing of the area overstimulates the same area of the brain with normal stimulus. By doing this, you override the initial pain stimulus, and the result is that you perceive less pain. The shin is still bruised, maybe bleeding, but the brain is perceiving normality[196].

Similarly, there is the example of lower back pain for a few weeks from an inflamed joint. Every time you put weight through that joint, a specific part of your brain is stimulated, and you experience pain. My job is to provide the normal stimulus again, except that instead of rubbing the joint, we can offer a movement stimulus in the form of muscle releases and adjustments.

---

[195] I attribute the inspiration of some of the topics here to Dr Dan Murphy, someone who I believe is one of the most brilliant medical minds in the world. I have applied his teachings to my own life and in my practice.

[196] This, in a nutshell, is why you feel *so* good after having your neck and back cracked. There is some science behind the feel-good feeling. Endorphins are released and the signal to the brain is a signal of normal movement again. Any pain from the joint, (from inflammation or the joint being stuck), is overridden and you feel *good*.

If we can move the said painful joint, we override the perceived painful memory. We literally teach the body that it is okay to move that joint. What normally happens is that by the next day the brain can still perceive the same pain, but it will often be less severe. So, we move the joint again. And again. Eventually the body recognises the normal movement.

You can see that this process takes longer than pain killers, but the long-term, essential benefit from restoring normal movement removes the need for pain killers altogether.

Zone 2 Exercise

Exercise alone has an anti-inflammatory effect, but where I see exercise being most beneficial is in maintaining normal joint movement, increasing blood flow and strengthening the neuromusculoskeletal memory. As you have just seen from the gate control mechanism, the right kind of exercise will overload the nervous system with positive and pain-free stimulus, and if I have observed one thing that exercise does for me, it is that it creates a craving. The body craves the good feeling of being pain free. As previously mentioned, endorphins and cannabinoids combat pain, and these are released during exercise.

Omega 3 vs Omega 6 Ratio

If you want to take one supplement for your pain, take Omega 3 oils. A ratio that favours Omega 6 is shown to increase inflammation in the body. When there is too much inflammation in the body, the signals to the central nervous system are altered, adding to the perceived pain.

Other beneficial supplements, some of which we became acquainted with in the previous chapter are Vitamin D, Resveratrol (100mg/day), Curcumin (200mg/day), Malic acid (2400mg/day), Magnesium (600mg/day), Antioxidants, Acetyl-l-carnitine, Alpha-lipoic acid, Coenzyme Q10.

Hot or Cold

I always get asked which is better. Hot or cold. My answer, every time, is that either of them is better than doing nothing. That is my inner optimist coming out.

The whole reason you put extreme temperature on your injury or body part is to increase blood flow. There are other cellular level changes that happen but the science behind it lies in the stimulation of blood flow. Always remember, both need to be on for longer than seven minutes to elicit a therapeutic response.

Take both scenarios. As you put an ice pack on your skin, the body freaks out and immediately vasoconstricts (narrows or closes) all the blood vessels in the area. It does this so that you will not lose heat. The body's natural response will be to direct blood away from the area. You can observe this by the paleness of the area if you remove the ice during this time. The ice will also be painful for the first three minutes. Very painful[197]. After around three minutes of having an ice pack on your skin, your body will now vasodilate (open the blood vessels), and allow your body to try and heat the area, because now there is a risk of damaging cells as the result of the cold. Again, this is easily observed. If you remove the ice after

---

[197] Do you remember Jack Dawson in the movie TITANIC? Jack was explaining to Rose how water, as cold as iceberg water, hits you like a thousand knives, stabbing you all over your body. You cannot breathe. You cannot think. If you have not experienced an ice bath yet, please try it. Or even just a cold shower is beneficial. Either way, you will hate me for it, but you will feel amazing afterwards.

around seven minutes, the area where the pack was is now red. This means blood has rushed to the area.

At the other end of the spectrum we have heat. As you put a heat pack or hot water bottle on your skin, the body reacts similarly to the way it did with the ice pack, except that it immediately vasodilates all the blood vessels in the area. It does this so that we will absorb heat. The body's natural response will be to direct blood towards the area. You can observe this by the redness of the area if you remove the heat during this time. Again, after around three minutes of having the heat pack on your skin, the body will now vasoconstrict as the body is now at risk of damaging cells because of the heat.

After seven minutes of either, there is now new blood in the area. This is important to understand. Before the ice or heat, the area would have had some form of protective spasm, especially if there was pain experienced in the area or simply inflammation without a sensation of pain.

The thing about spasm is that there would have been restricted movement in the area for some time, and this would have decreased blood flow to the area. When there is decreased blood flow, the waste products of normal metabolism build up, these are called Metabolites. There is thus an increased pressure in the blood system in the injured area. The crux here is to understand that blood flow goes only from arteries to tissues and then to veins or lymph drainage (the extra bits). Blood cannot flow in the opposite direction. Whether you have used ice or heat, once blood has been pushed out of the area, only new blood can flow into it. New blood brings oxygen and all the good cells needed to heal the area, less the metabolites.

Now imagine if you alternated ice and then heat, or vice versa. More blood turnover means faster healing. This does not only apply to injuries. It can be used preventatively too. It can speed up your recovery from exercise. It can increase circulation in the elderly. It can make you feel like a professional athlete.

I treat many people over the age of 60. With age, the body becomes biased with its own blood, and with that, healing slows down. The most practical way I explain this to elderly patients is to say that the body keeps the blood circulating to the brain and all the organs, and it slows down the periphery blood circulation to your arms and legs.

I remember vividly my grandfather, aged 75 at the time, having an ulcer on his leg from a small procedure that had been performed on his leg. That hole next to his tibia took months to heal, purely because blood flow was slowed, and blood is what brings all the healing agents. That is why I strongly advise using ice and heat therapy to drastically speed up the healing process, which, in turn, affects the pain process.

Point to ponder: Are you tired of taking pain medication? If so, the best pain relief is reminding the body what normal feels like.

Natural Pain Management

HOLISTIC PAIN MANAGEMENT STRATEGY	HOW IT HELPS YOUR PAIN
Gate control theory or Neural Re-education (NRE)	Non-painful sensation overrides painful sensation which prevents the painful sensation from traveling to the brain
Zone 2 exercise	Decreases inflammation Releases endorphins, endocannabinoids Stops the stress/ cortisol cycle Helps insulin resistance[198]
Heat application	Increases blood flow to speed up healing Decreases inflammation Relaxes muscle spasm
Cold application	After reducing blood flow, blood flow increases Decreases inflammation
Omega 3 vs Omega 6 ratio (More Omega 3)	Decreases inflammation
Vitamin D	Decreases inflammation
Clean eating	Decreases inflammation Helps insulin resistance
Avoid foods containing glutamate and aspartate	Creates chronic pain sensitization
Stop smoking	Decreases pain sensation

---

[198] Pain and insulin resistance seem to be in bed together. You are welcome to browse the reference list to see just how intimate they are.

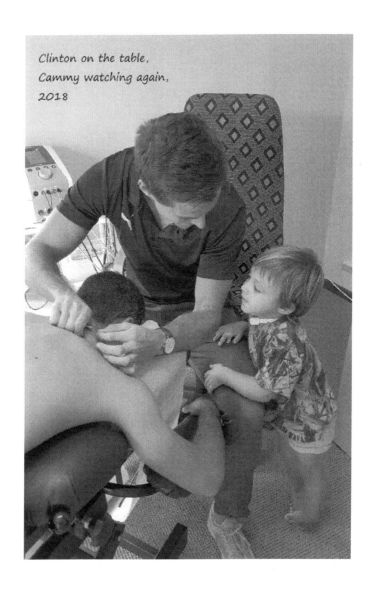

Clinton on the table,
Cammy watching again,
2018

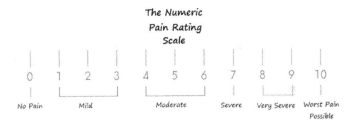

The Numeric
Pain Rating
Scale

0   1   2   3   4   5   6   7   8   9   10

No Pain   Mild   Moderate   Severe   Very Severe   Worst Pain
                                                            Possible

19 : Healing

Jon's treatment: NRE protocol. Release muscle tension QL's and deep Glutes. Traction using bed manual traction and mechanical drop pieces. Adjust the pelvis below and the spine above lesion site. Heat therapy at home. Encourage movement within pain ranges. Let the disc breathe a bit.

There is no "I" in *health*, but there is "heal". Here is my saying again. Healing is not rocket science. You create the environment to heal, and you will heal. If you do not make time for your wellness, you will be forced to make time for your illness. Healing is not a *have to*, it is a *get to*. You get to change the trajectory of where your health is headed. I believe that is not something we should take for granted.

Let us not fool ourselves, there is no quick way of doing this. The day you plant the seed is not the day you enjoy the fruit. Our minds cannot be happy if our bodies are not free from suffering. Before we can diagnose anyone, we need to make sure there is no sickness in the mind or the heart. Therefore, this is the foremost step, answering the question *where is your mind at?*

The First Step: Choice

As a patient you need to be expectant of healing. If you do not believe that our minds and emotions have influence over us to some degree, look at someone who is in love. Listen to how their stomachs rumble, as they experience butterflies. Some emotions cannot be explained by science, they really are mind over matter. And for this reason, the first step towards becoming healthy is making a choice.

If you want to know how strong the mind is, look at your biology. Have you ever thought just how incredible dreams are? Your mind literally enters a different reality. So powerful that you can have a physiological reaction from your mind and imagination. An example of is that of a 'wet dream', how the body can experience a full sexual orgasm, purely from an experience in your mind. Think of nightmares that cause full body sweats. And consider sleep walking; how a six-year-old boy can take a 25kg bag of firewood to bed with him, yet when he is awake and conscious there would be no chance that he would do that[199]. That is the power of the mind. And the power of mind over *perceived* matter.

---

[199] This is a true story. It concerns my cousin Tyler. I have friends who sleepwalk, others I know sleep talk and even some who sleep stalk. Thinking about it now, the latter is probably something they should have checked out psychologically.

The 2016 film "Split" follows the unravelling of a man suffering from a dissociative identity disorder. Kevin, played by James McAvoy, has 23 alter egos. He, (or they), end(s) up kidnapping a few teenagers. The movie explores how the hostages must figure out his friendly personas before he unleashes his 24th personality. The elusive 24th persona, called the *Beast*, emerges in all its glory, as an amalgam of Kevin's qualities, and the highest form of physical human advancement.

Hollywood aside, in real life the physical changes that occur in a switch between alter egos is one of the most baffling aspects of dissociative identity disorder. Patients can assume whole new physical postures and voices and vocabularies. And I believe I have seen this in practice.

Here is an example.

June 2019

Tony Soprano, a 52-year-old male patient presents to the clinic. Patient explains he battles to balance his family life.

Tony presented with mild mechanical-related low back pain and mentioned that he feels that some days he has a shorter leg (today was one of those days). He has a previously diagnosed dissociative identity disorder - in this case bipolar.

We perform a few Waddell's signs, (theses are tests to see if a patient is faking their symptoms. Yes, these are real), and we rule out Alice in Wonderland Syndrome and Alien Hand Syndrome (I honestly wish I could make some of these conditions up!).

X-rays were justified and taken. Tony had a significant structural S-shaped scoliosis, more than seven degrees both ways[200]. It makes sense that the leg length functional tests that day were irregular. It makes sense that Tony experienced a shorter leg.

We began a NRE protocol and something bizarre happened over the next few months. Every time I saw the patient, his leg length was different, and stories from the previous week did not correlate.

New X-rays were justified and taken after six weeks. The new X-rays showed that the spine was almost dead straight.

The good-to-knows:

ONE. I have treated many patients; this one is a near impossibility. It is almost miraculous. A curve that severe simply cannot correct in six weeks. It does not make clinical, practical, possible, or logical sense. It was either a miracle or his body physically changed with his alter egos. Perhaps one day we will find an ethical approach to clinically studying this type of case.

TWO. I have seen hundreds of scoliosis patients and they never responded this well or this quickly, and certainly not this structurally.

THREE. I wish we could X-ray him at every treatment and see exactly what happened, but I may lose my professional registration for over-radiating a patient. Nevertheless, there is evidence that we should never underestimate the power of the mind.

---

[200] Functional scoliosis (meaning the spine is curved secondary to other factors like muscle imbalances or heavy school bags) normally respond well to treatment, whereas with most structural scoliosis, (meaning that the bones have physically changed shape as in Mr Soprano's case), you cannot decrease the curve at all. In those cases, you manage the symptoms and prevent the curve from getting worse. Telling a patient that is in no way negative. It depends how you see it. Is the cup half empty or half full? *Mindset.*

Internal Healing Environment

You have heard these words a few times now. Let us take it a little deeper. The body is designed to heal itself. Within the correct internal environment, the immune system, which is controlled by the nervous system, will provide the ultimate medium for cellular regeneration and repair. You could call this natural healing or wellness and there is currently a global trend towards it.

Healing is multifaceted, complex and counter-cultural. The internal environment will select the genetic activity of every cell replication. A healing environment leads to perfect replication. A stressed environment leads to potential alterations. We have seen this already in *Little Soix* chapter.

If you give the body what it needs, it will heal. This includes enough sleep, water, clean eating and exercise. It also benefits from hopeful, positive and loving thoughts and feelings. Fear, anxiety, stress, and apathy are the enemies of wellness. Shift your perspective to a more relaxed and confident state of mind. This promotes healing.

While it is not always easy to make time for yourself, self-care is the cornerstone of healing and health. Our busy lifestyles do not encourage putting ourselves first, which is absurd. If we do not take good care of ourselves, who will? We need to try creating more *me* time, to make time to exercise but also to relax, pray, read, pamper, write and do whatever we find joy in. Maybe that means travelling - if you have the means to travel. Your body will reward you. Remember to *put your oxygen mask on first.*

There is no quick fix. There are no magic remedies. There is no genie offering wishes. Healing takes time and discipline at first, but eventually it becomes habitual and normal. No one can heal you, but yourself. Modern medicine may lessen symptoms, or even make them *go away* for a short while, but that is not the same as healing. The same imbalances will still exist, and another set of symptoms will appear down the road until you take charge of your health, and tune in to your body, mind and spirit to make any changes needed.

The Second Step: Discipline

It is only the disciplined ones who experience freedom; do not become a slave to your emotions[201]. Building healthy habits is a transformation that takes both consistency and discipline. You may need to choose to be healthy many times throughout your day, and it may not always feel good immediately, but sometimes we need to do what we must, to do what we want.

So, how exactly can a disciplined lifestyle improve healing? The answer is related to the fact that stress *can* literally kill you. Now, I see and manage many stressed patients[202]. When your body is stressed it releases a hormone called cortisol via the hypothalamus pituitary adrenal axis. In small doses, cortisol is marvellous! It is almost euphoric - a fight or flight hormone. Imagine you come across a lion in the Serengeti. You either fight it or you run away from it. Cortisol prepares the body for that.

---

[201] Fight the urges to eat your feelings. Do not have sweet stuff in your house, this way you are less likely to *stress eat*. Do not let thoughts like 'I am not in the mood to go for a run' overthrow your healthy desires. We teach the body these good habits, when you are feeling demotivated and lazy, do exercise, force a 30 min walk at least, and you will have more energy afterwards having burnt some. Eventually your body craves this feeling. Until then, sometimes you just *gotta fake it 'til ya make it*.

[202] This sounds impossible but you can *see* stress in someone. Their shoulders do not have fluidity as a result of all the physical tension. There is a distinct frown line between the eyes, a subconscious worry. There is a slump in their demeanour, in other words their posture depresses, and there is an obvious lack of sleep. The breathing rhythm is laboured, and there is a tendency to sweat more than normal or have a nervous twitch. There is increased smoking and/or drinking, and the consumption of too many unhealthy foods. The other extreme is having no appetite. These are all tell-tale signs of stress.

This is not so great when your body prepares for that choice while you are sitting at your desk. Most likely, before your workday officially starts, your body starts secreting cortisol out of your adrenal gland. Chronic cortisol can disrupt almost all of your body's natural processes, and in turn, increase your chances of many health problems. Therefore, daily stress needs to be counteracted.

How can you re-teach your body to not prepare for stress at the beginning of the workday? And how can you stress less? Well, it is simple, although harder than it sounds.

Not many people can snap out of *stress* in a heartbeat. The most practical way of going about counteracting stress would be regularly *breaking* the cycle of it. We have already seen how exercise does this, how clean eating can aid it, but we must not underestimate the hourly mini breaks. The act of leaving your workstation, taking a few deep breaths, stretching through a doorway, swinging your legs, doing a squat followed by a twist, drinking some water, and returning to your workstation, are all examples of mini breaks. Physically, mentally and emotionally, the stress cycle will temporarily halt. Many halts eventually become a habit.

Think again of the analogy of a seesaw. Stress is the opposite of healing. Too much stress and the body cannot attain an internal healing environment. Stress opposes health. Stress promotes injury and illness. There needs to be the right cocktail of recovery and diet along with flexibility, improvement, core strength and balance exercises.

The main thing to remember here is that you need to take baby steps and be patient, or you may become one.

343

The Third Step: Attitude

I always know during the case history part of the consultation, pretty much within the first ten minutes of meeting someone, whether they will respond well to treatment or not. And that has to do with their attitude and mindset towards wanting to get better. Most healing happens because there is a healthy environment in which it can occur. Some patients' attitudes put a real limitation on the extent to which I can help them. Further education and counselling are needed in those cases.

Healing is optimized when the patient is emotionally grounded in intentions to heal and to be healed. Healing is fostered by inner beliefs and expectations that healing and wellness can and will occur. My cousin Don from earlier, who survived cancer, is one of the thousands of patients I have seen who remind me of the authenticity of this.

Be Expectant

This attitude or internal environment of *being expectant* consists of our most private thoughts, hopes, emotions, intentions, and beliefs. Understanding each dimension and the interdependence of the mind, body, and spirit are crucial to health creation and healing.

Expectation is the conscious thought of being expectant to getting better. We saw in the chapter *Your First Time* that often the likelihood of a patient responding to our treatment is often determined by their attitude. I emphasize the word often numerous times because there are millions of exceptions to this rule.

Have you heard of the *Rosenthal Effect*? If not, it is worth a google search. Long story short, the Rosenthal Effect is a psychological phenomenon wherein high expectations lead to improved performance in a given area. When someone expects a given result, that expectation unconsciously affects the outcome.

I believe that I have witnessed this phenomenon, both from the patient's side and from the doctor's side. Positive expectation gives us a lot of power, both as a patient and as a doctor. The positive feedback effect of an expectant doctor is as powerful as the positive feedback effect of an expectant patient.

When your doctor tells you there is no hope, there is a massive chance you will not get better. When a patient tells me there is no hope, I try my hardest to change their perspective, because I know that there is a massive chance that they will not get better without it. Many times I have told patients indirectly that there is no hope of full recovery which is the reality sometimes, but in the same breath I have made it clear that there is always something to improve; there is always something positive to take out, and there is always a way to get them moving to the best of their ability. This is the important take-away here - there is always room for improvement, and it is never too late[203].

Without overthinking this aspect or delving in too deeply, our attitude is vital to healing because our mindset has a direct effect on our bodies, our choices, and our relationships. And all of those are needed to heal.

---

[203] I see this every day when patients tell me what they have previously been diagnosed with something, and how it is evident that the diagnosis has affected their entire outlook on life. I believe the desires of the doctor have a part to play in the outcome of the patient's response. If your doctor genuinely wants to help you get better (greater than their desire to make money), then the likelihood of them helping you is enormous. Maybe one day they will name this health phenomenon the *Cuan effect*.

The Last Step: Relationships

We have already seen how having a support system around you makes your recovery process vastly more efficient. One form of support is joining in this journey with your health care practitioner, whoever it may be. *We do it together.*

As a Health Coach and chiropractor, I can facilitate the healing process to some degree as follows.

ONE. Physically, by restoring normal movement, through *Neural Re-Education* and by educating the brain concerning what normal joint and muscle movements should feel like. Also, physically, by promoting exercise and by taking physical stressors off the autonomic nervous system[204].

TWO. Emotionally, by offering emotional support and guiding belief towards encouraging optimism, along with stress management and helping a patient cope with the stressors of life.

THREE. Chemically, by encouraging eating clean. By trying to identify dietary stressors and offering dietary advice.

FOUR. Psychologically, by motivating patients.

FIVE. Spiritually, helping patients believe, if not in something bigger than themselves, then in themselves.

---

[204] There are textbooks on the autonomic nervous system. All you need to know is that the autonomic nervous system is the part of our nervous system which is responsible for placing us in a healing environment. This is also the part of the nervous system that can be affected by adjusting (cracking) the spine. When you understand that the brain and nervous system control everything in your body, you should feel *psyched-up* to have regular check-ups.

The Power of Patience

You heard from a friend of mine earlier - Bradley Birkholtz. He is a real-life example of this. Brad is one of the fastest amateur triathletes in the world. I asked him if he would be willing to write a testimony and here it is[205].

Cuan always told me that the body will heal itself, you just need to be patient. You need to believe in the process. When you are injured, do not aggravate the injury further by stressing it more and training on it. When I recall the world championships, I remember that I had a serious injury. It was seriously painful. We had a couple of treatments and eventually we agreed that I would not run for two weeks before the world championships. We agreed that I would rather give myself a fighting chance at getting to the start line, and even if the injury flared up during the race, at least I would be racing. And it did flare up during the last three or four kilometres, but I had enough grit to carry me through and I ended up running a personal best time. It was unbelievable.

Cuan always said that the treatment will work, but that you need to be patient. And that is something you learn only with experience. We all want overnight fixes. When patience is key, the body will heal. Knowing that your treatment aids that process speeds it along. The body knows what it should do.

One example I remember is when he described how needling causes a trauma and sends good blood to the injury to promote healing. This takes time. In a way you are creating an injury to improve the injury.

He has also always advocated stretching, stretching, stretching. Proprioception. Getting used to mobility exercises should not be something you do as part of recovery days; it should be a daily lifestyle thing. I have even changed the way I sit at work and I take regular breaks. I also add regular stretches to my work hours. This is especially important for

---

[205] I wish I could have paid him to say these things because they are so spot on.

runners who are pounding away at the body every day.

I have been lucky not to have had many injuries, and I think a lot of that is because I have learnt from Cuan how to manage my body. I do not run on too many consecutive days. I prioritize Zone 2 sessions. I also make time for stretching. And, when there is a hint of an injury, I back off a bit and stay patient.

The only other thing I would add is to say he taught me confidence in what I do and confidence in the process. As an athlete you understand what goes through another athlete's mind. I remember when he diagnosed my ankle as a bad grade 2 tear, and two months after that injury I was still in pain. I was considering surgery, but he told me to be patient, and trust the system. And I remember, just like that, one day it was perfect again.

Point to ponder: Have you done something to help create a healing environment today?

TYPES OF SCOLIOSIS OF SPINE

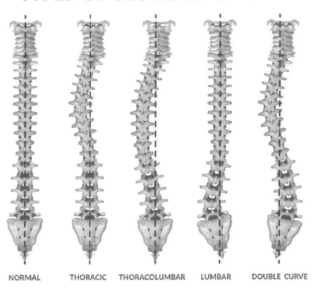

NORMAL   THORACIC   THORACOLUMBAR   LUMBAR   DOUBLE CURVE

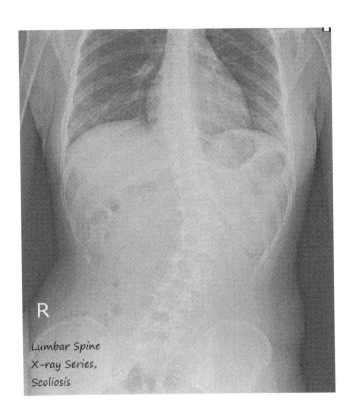

R

Lumbar Spine
X-ray Series,
Scoliosis

20 : The *F-word*

Jon's prognosis: Pain drastically decreased in 3 - 6 treatments (if not, refer a.s.a.p.). Full function in 6 weeks. Following rehab program, running in 3 months. Suspect full recovery. *Maths.*

S ometimes it seems to me that chiropractic in the public mind is regarded as a blasphemy of some kind. Voodoo. Health care by quacks. (Fake doctors, as you read earlier). I thought it would only make sense to give some history to my profession of choice and why I practise as I do. As with any health care field, there are different styles of chiropractic. I rarely even call myself a chiropractor anymore. I practice as a chiropractor, but I prefer the term *Health*

Coach[206].

Digital marketing these days presents all sorts of magic remedies, drugs, or treatments that will cure all in no time. Instead of spending money on too-good-to-be-true medicines, there is so much you can do for yourself (mostly free) in the form of clean eating and moving your body in the way it was designed to move. The result is optimum health since the body is self-healing. Invest time in yourself. If advocating a health philosophy such as this one makes me a 'quack', then that I am.

Chiropractic

Chiropractic literally means *hand practice*; that is to have a health care practice where your only tool for healing is your hands. While I was travelling in Israel in 2019, I joked with our tour guide that Jesus must have been the first chiropractor as He healed with His hands. I do appreciate a sense of humour in times like that. The truth is that some of the cases I have witnessed and been lucky enough to be a part of, are nothing short of miracles.

The founder of chiropractic was DD Palmer in 1895. After his death in 1913, a century of conflict followed between the *straights* and the *mixers* regarding how to define chiropractic health care. Palmer wrote, "No, thank you, I do not mix. I give chiropractic *straight*." I can imagine him saying to me "*It is my way or the highway!*".

---

[206] There is a practical joke among chiropractors that you are not a real chiropractor until you have cracked someone's rib. This is an extremely rare but possible adverse effect of pushing someone into a firm chiropractic bed. Therefore, it is more beneficial to use different techniques for the middle back like standing or seated mobilizations. The point of this story is that I guess I am not a *real* chiropractor anyway.

The *straights* defined chiropractic as focused on the analysis and correction of the vertebral subluxation, (the joint misalignment), the cause of all health problems, to foster the fullest expression of the individual's innate intelligence. If you read that last sentence again, and if it does not make sense to you at first glance, then join the club, that is a normal feeling at first. This is one reason that the medical fraternity dislikes chiropractors in general. You heard earlier how Dr Spring, a medical doctor and gynaecologist, was sceptical to even see me as my patient at first, and I completely understand why. Anyone with a scientific brain will not like hearing things like *"I let innate tell me which joint to adjust"*.

The S-word

To try and explain that in more simple terms, *straight* chiropractors believe that the vertebral subluxation, or the *S-word*, causse all illness. They believe that an internal force called *"innate"* controls everything. The claim is that they do not diagnose or treat disease, rather they remove the subluxations and let innate express health in the body.

You can see how different that description of chiropractic is compared to this entire book so far.

Here is my point. Some of my *straight* colleagues are the most effective healers I know. This speaks to the importance of belief, attitude and relationships, as we saw in the previous chapter. Within the healing chapter we saw that the first step of healing is a choice. If you trust and believe that you can heal, chances are you will. If you trust and believe that your practitioner will help you heal, he or she *most likely* will.

Health Coach

I have always practiced as a *mixer*. By *mixer* I mean that I define chiropractic more broadly - as I have done in this book. As a chiropractor, I practice as a health coach.

In South Africa, the chiropractic degree is mechanistic, more medical- and evidence-based. I even used my brother's medical textbooks for the first three years of my chiropractic degree. Anatomy, physiology, pharmacology, pathology to name a few[207].

In dealings with medical doctors, I have regularly noticed that there is always a preconceived idea of what I do. When I started practice, I did take offense to some of the 'banter'. It felt as if it was my duty to correct the perception that the medical doctors had. However, this idea that I needed to change their bias quickly went away. I learnt that it was important to let my actions speak for me. Within a few months, I had treated a handful of doctors after they were referred to me by their own patients. These doctors, in turn, started referring other patients of their own. One of the best descriptions of what I do was given by a patient of mine who referred someone to me. "If you want an answer to your issue" they said, "see Cuan". Finding the answer - understanding the cause - solving the problem. Ultimately, that is what I do, I am a problem solver, also known as a health coach.

You have just read about pain and about healing in recent chapters. The common denominator is that both are related to

---

[207] I told you earlier about the second time I was kicked out of class. The first time was an anatomy-related event. After two years of having the same cadaver to work on, we were required to present our findings to the class in the form of a PowerPoint presentation. In other words, every group summarised our anatomy textbook, it was rather boring. My group had other plans. We made a music video involving our cadaver. After playing it for the class, we stood there expecting a standing ovation. Instead we were met with *dead* silence. (Excuse the pun.) We were immediately asked to leave and had to offer a formal apology.

your brain[208]. The reason I prefer the term *health coach* is that there is no *one answer* for what a health coach does, but the goal is the same, to get your body into a healing environment, to tilt the seesaw in healing's favour. The body can heal itself if we attain this.

My role is to direct your attitude towards wanting to heal and simply to help you to be the best version of yourself. Your journey of healing begins with a conscious choice and ends with the act of a recovery-driven lifestyle.

My role is to form a relationship and to journey with you. From my experience, this relationship always contains some clean eating. The relationship always contains some Zone 2 exercise. And it always contains excessive education.

My role includes physical treatment. This treatment needs to be condition- and patient-specific. There is no single treatment for all. There are too many tools of my trade to mention here, but the frequently used ones I find most advantageous hands-on are: stretching, trigger point release, dry needling, acupuncture, and joint mobilisations.

My role goes beyond the symptomatic improvement of local tissues. Treatment should not be pain-based alone, although, feeling good is a by-product. That said, pain relief is often the patient's main objective. In these cases, my role is to do whatever is needed to decrease your pain or prevent it from coming back. Refer to the chapter on *Pain.*

My role is to identify the environment that is preventing you from excelling at health. We walk that journey together. We do not only want to get you back to your previous health - we would like to get you better than before.

Can you live without something like this? *Of course.*

Could you live better with something like this? *Oh yes.*

I love this summary below, written by Dr Robyn Spring, the

---

[208] Remember, pain is literally in the brain. Pain is a perception. Pain is an experience. We can re-educate the brain to know what non-painful experiences are. And this is exciting!

gynaecologist you met earlier in the Chapter *Core, Back Pain and Pregnancy*. This is not blowing my own trumpet; this is NOT about me. Wherever you see *Cuan*, replace that with any of one my likeminded colleagues. By likeminded colleagues I mean anyone, from any profession, who puts a patient's needs first.

I first met Cuan rather reluctantly, since as a conventionally trained doctor, one is trained to view some allied health practitioners with suspicion. However, to my absolute joy, I found him to be professional, accurate and realistic in his approach. He had correctly identified several running injuries I had developed, identified the reason they had developed and prescribed a comprehensive rehabilitation plan. After this I have been able to run marathons, ultra-marathons and multiday trail events in good condition. Unfortunately, he did not have a magic wand to make me run faster and podium, but that is forgiven by the mere fact that I run pain-free and happy now. Without a shadow of doubt, an encounter with Cuan has changed my running fortune forever.

I am grateful for having had the privilege to work alongside Dr Spring. Someone else who I am also blessed to have worked with is Dr Jason Thoresen.

The F-word

We have covered many different conditions in this book already, I would like to draw your attention to one more, Fibromyalgia. Or the *F-word*. This is a chronic pain syndrome with no known cause. In other words, a patient experiences widespread musculoskeletal pain accompanied by fatigue, sleep, memory and mood issues, and the cause is said to be unknown, or *idiopathic*[209].

Why I view it as the *F-word* is because more often than not it is used in contexts where it is not necessary, and it is often used in the place of a word we cannot think of at the time. In other words, fibromyalgia diagnoses are at times not necessary or merely done so in the absence of an alternative answer.

I worked in East London (South Africa) for seven years. During this time, I practiced from a family medical centre. This was an important time of growth for me. It was here that I would practice and develop into what kind of practitioner I wanted to be. It was also here that I had the joy of working with one of the most thorough medical doctors that I know, Dr Thoresen.

Between the two of us, we had witnessed numerous cases of diagnosed *F-words* that responded extremely well to our treatment approach[210]. Over four years of consciously referring fibromyalgia patients between the two of us, we found we were able to help upward of ninety percent of these cases. In my opinion, all we did was sort out the mechanics, and their bodies did the rest.

Here is a summary of our findings, written by Dr Thoresen.
Over the last four years, since I have been in private

---

[209] Dr House from the tv series House said it best: *Idiopathic*, from the Latin, meaning we are idiots because we cannot figure out what is causing it.

[210] Please understand that this is counter-cultural to popular belief. Results are not normally positive. On paper fibromyalgia and all the chronic pain syndromes are a sad diagnosis with no reported treatment.

practice, Cuan and I have worked together in the same building, Famcare, in East London. I started seeing numerous patients who had previously been diagnosed with fibromyalgia and who had subsequently been put on chronic medication for this diagnosis. No underlying risk factors were ever identified. I wanted to see what common underlying pathology I could identify and treat to get these patients off their chronic medications. It was evident that the medications were only masking the symptoms of the chronic pain syndrome.

After I investigated and enquired further, and looked at the patient's histories, it appeared that most of the cases had some sort of back pathology, back pain or back complaint. Many these cases had previous spinal surgeries. Going forward, I hypothesized that there must be a link between the spine and these fibromyalgia cases.

This was where Cuan came in. In chatting with him, he said that he regularly had patients with previous fibromyalgia diagnoses who responded to his treatments. I found this bizarre as all the medical literature speaks about this condition as having no successful treatment options. But Cuan's claims made sense IF there was a link between the spine and this condition's clinical presentation.

As an unofficial trial, I found 10 patients who were already visiting our practice. These patients were already on medical therapy like antidepressants, antianxiety medications, and other medications known to help with neurological pain conduction. All the patients had a pain rating of above 7/10 daily. Patients without existing spinal x-rays were sent for x-ray investigations. The x-ray findings were unanimous, and we observed arthritic and spondylitic changes evident of degenerative processes occurring within the spine.

I referred these patients to Cuan for a trial of conservative treatment including spinal adjustments and physical therapy. 9 out of the 10 patients responded in terms of pain rating and overall activity of daily living. 1 of the 10 patients did not respond (which I believed to be as a result of severe and pre-

existing depression).

This trial opened a whole new thinking process to medicine and treating patients with chronic pain syndromes. We concluded that there is a big opening in terms of first-line treatment recommendations, especially for Fibromyalgia. This does NOT mean that patients should stop their medications immediately, or at all. It is merely a new thinking strategy to some of the alternative options which are effective. Approaches from GPs need to be updated where physical therapy should be at least mentioned to a patient before commencement of chronic and often addictive pain medications.

Dr Thoreson and I wanted to try publishing this information in the form of a journal article. We were both too busy at the time. So, this is the first step to that, or merely a step in educating the public.

Everything we did and advised to the patients was covered in the pain management chapter.

It also helped drastically that we took time to educate the patients and let them ask questions. In most fibromyalgia cases that I have seen myself, the patients have described consultations where no tests have been conducted, yet this diagnosis is often thrown around. It seems it is often a case of diagnosis by exclusion. What I am trying to reiterate, is that education and accurate diagnosis are often lost in the current systems.

If you think that this could have applied in your treatment, obtain a second, third or fourth opinion.

The message here is that very often, this and many other sad diagnoses end up causing widespread destruction. Most patients suffering from chronic pain syndromes are on anti-depressant medications. Most of them walk into our rooms and the biggest battle we have is getting them to believe that something *can* be done for them. Once they choose to try help themselves, the good fight begins. The *F-word* changes its meaning to Freedom.

Freedom from pain.

This is the basis for a holistic approach. There is rarely a single cause for a chronic ailment. You need to identify every aspect that is adding to the internal lack of healing in the individual.

It was a privilege working with a doctor like Jason - someone who lives and breathes putting patients first. He was a catalyst in my personal motivation to always read up on the latest research. He reminded me that knowledge is power in our fields. And in turn I learnt that this knowledge meant I could serve people better.

Until we work together again[211].

---

[211] Raises a glass with Dr T. I hope that this is a spoiler for the future.

Point to ponder: What is the *F-word* in your
life and maybe there is a way to turn it around?

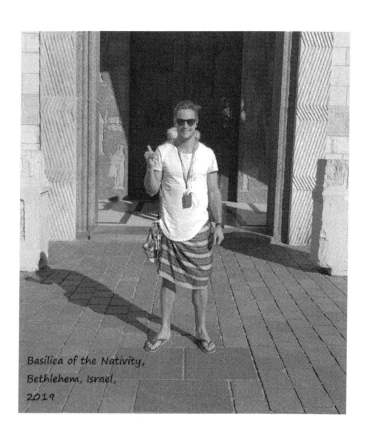

Basilica of the Nativity,
Bethlehem, Israel,
2019

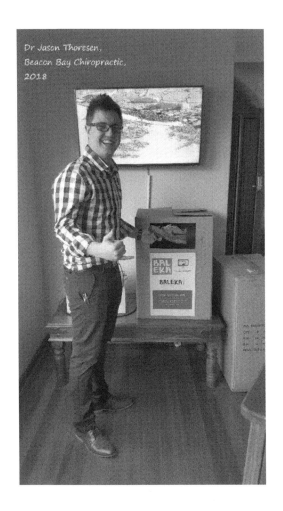

Dr Jason Thoresen,
Beacon Bay Chiropractic,
2018

21 : Your Move

Jon does not want treatment and leaves the practice.

The health philosophy I have shared with you in these pages through anecdote and experience, is about interrogating the way we view health and health care. Over the years, I have observed a medical system that is set up to treat disease whilst failing to encourage wellness. I have found that there is no more potent or effective medicine than exercise and clean eating.

Forget the thought of making a change when it is a convenient time. That will NEVER come. There is no need to wait and every reason not to, especially in stressful times.

I have learnt so much about myself from dealings with thousands of patients who have all granted me the privilege of meeting and managing their health goals with them. What every one of them has taught me is that if you put the effort in, you will get the results out.

Here are some last-minute thoughts:
ONE. Consistency is key. Consistency leads to a compound effect. If you know money, you know the value of compounding interest. I tell this to all my athletes, and it is the same principle with your health. Try to limit the bad days.
TWO. If you think that your health is sublime, and you do not need a tune-up, remember, even a Ferrari needs one.
THREE. You cannot build a foundation without digging a hole. If your health has dug a hole in recent years, you have all the potential to make a change. The good thing about being rock-bottom is that there is only *upwards* from there.
FOUR. The most important attribute I have witnessed in patients who respond favourably to treatment is a positive attitude.

Jon Snow

Regarding Jon Snow's case that you have followed throughout the book.

The ONE good-to-know is this: You can take a horse to the water, but you cannot make it drink. In real life, it may kick you.

The mere fact that this book is in your hand means you are positioned to make an informed decision. The next step requires you to act on it. One conscious move towards transforming your life.

Why Move at All?

Now that I have hopefully got you thinking about a few novel changes you might make in the way that you care for yourself or understand health care, I need to go deeper and ask why any of it matters in the first place? To what end does one seek a healthy lifestyle that promotes longevity? We are all only on this earth for a limited time, and we do not seem to get to be here exceedingly long. Some lose their lives before they even begin. Others are cut short. It is a stark realisation when we lose a loved one - that even forever with them would not have felt long enough. It therefore makes sense to me that we use the years we do have to live out a life of purpose and being healthy grants us the freedom to live out that purpose most effectively.

Speaking about what you believe can always feel a bit tricky. It feels like tippy toeing around an angry sleeping bear. I will therefore endeavour to tippy toe as I share with you some fundamental revelations that motivate what I do and give meaning to my pursuit of health and my provision of health care.

Firstly, I know why I get up every morning, I know who I am and most importantly, I know *whose* I am. My identity is defined internally by believing in God and knowing that Jesus died so that I may have a relationship with Him. I believe insecurities come from not having your identity in something bigger than yourself.

Secondly, I know that there will be times of barrenness and destruction. Times when things are not going well. Times of uncertainty and financial need. Times of heartache and mourning. Times when my nephew is on his death bed. Times when all seems lost. I know from experience that the storms of life will come, and that no matter how alone, angry and hurt I feel at the time, that I will get through it, and I won't have to do it alone. We all have bad days and feel hopeless at times - it is on these days that I remind myself of 'why' I need to pick myself up and carry on. *The sun always comes out eventually.*

Thirdly, loving God and loving others (yes, even the haters) is the only motivation I need to pour everything I am into helping my patients with their health needs. I hope that this passion for service to my patients is evident in this book and is evident if I ever treat you.

Finally, as someone currently alive, I am not scared to die. There is peace in knowing that my life is not my own, and that when my time here is up, I will have the honour to be with God for eternity. I try and serve my patients and serve God in such a way, that when I do get to be with the Lord one day, that He fist pumps me and utters the words, "You did good son and I am well pleased".

Sometimes, it is hard to see the bigger picture when you are stuck in the frame, so let us choose to get out, and have another look.

It is, and always has been, your move.

Point to ponder: Do not look back, are you
ready to make a move?

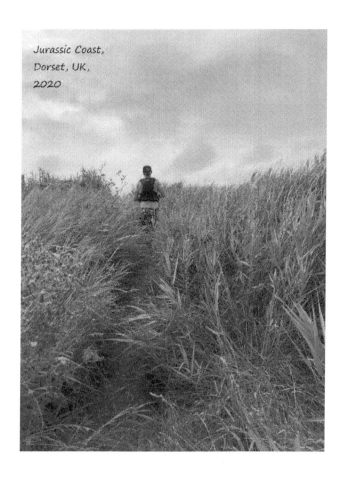

Jurassic Coast,
Dorset, UK,
2020

Epilogue

Cuan's Ten Commandments

COMMANDMENT #1: Thou shalt exercise and eat clean, for there is no greater medicine than this.

COMMANDMENT #2: Thou shalt not procrastinate or wait for a more convenient time, for such a time will not arrive.

COMMANDMENT #3: Thou shalt not corrupt thineself by taking shortcuts with thine health, for the effort thou puttest in doth, indeed, justify the means thou shalt benefit.

COMMANDMENT #4: Thou shalt always reap in direct proportion to how much thou hast sown.

COMMANDMENT #5: Thou shalt leave the world in a better condition than thou foundest it.

COMMANDMENT #6: Thou shalt leave the world's inhabitants happier than thou foundest them.

COMMANDMENT #7: Thou shalt strive for consistency, for it has a compound effect, and as the prophet Einstein foretold, "Compound interest is the 8th wonder of the world, and he who understands it shall earn it, and he who does not, shall pay it."

COMMANDMENT #8: Thou shalt not take thine health in vain - thou needest regular check-ups.

COMMANDMENT #9: Thou shalt only change if thou desirest change with all thine heart, soul, mind and strength.

COMMANDMENT #10: Thou, and thou alone, art responsible for the choices thou makest. Choose wisely, for thou shalt not move this way again.

Acknowledgements

Uncle Neil. You were my first and third editor. Your knowledge and input cannot be measured. I am grateful for your patience with me and with what originally was an extremely mislaid 'draft one'. Thank you.

Kerry. You were my second, fourth and final editor. I do not know how to thank you enough. Your ability to tell a story, that impacts everyone in it and those who read it, is a skill that cannot be taught. Besides transforming this book, you are a friend and an example to me to be gracious and to appreciate the process. Thank you.

Dan. The cover is a masterpiece. Classy and eloquent. Thank you.

More Eyewitnesses

Exemplary in all his endeavours, but especially in his field, Cuan makes a most credible author for this book! - Weyers Marais

It is a rare thing to encounter a gentleman of this calibre. Cuan is deeply motivated by a genuine desire to love God and faithfully serve Him. A natural leader and exhorter, his conviction to love others well is both humbling and admirable. He does nothing half-heartedly, but with guts and gusto. Anybody who has the privilege of journeying with this man will be greatly encouraged by witnessing his life, both professionally and personally. - Carl Pistorius

Cuan is chock-full of heart and has managed to spill this into his book. This book exudes inspiration, and not the 'pink and fluffy' unattainable kind. This is a most genuine and practical guide to a healthier and happier life. You will be left enriched and challenged, learning whilst laughing, all along the way. A very well-balanced view that is both insightful and funny! - Richard Simes

If you love life, don't waste time, for time is what life is made up of (Bruce lee). This always reminds me of Cuan, he managed to get the balance of life just right. - Dr Gregg Audie

It is difficult not to get caught up in Cuan's infectious passion! Whether for family, friends, faith, health or fitness, his enthusiasm and drive know no boundaries. It has been a privilege to experience his zest for life both personally and professionally. - Dr Jason Dicks

Having watched the unfolding career of Dr Coetzee for over a decade in both South Africa and the UK, he has a zest for life and brings an energy and enthusiasm to his profession. An energy one does not commonly find in peers of his generation. I wish him every success in fulfilling the enormous clinical potential he has to help his patients in the decades ahead. - Dr Ashton Vice

Three words come to mind when thinking about Cuan. Faith. Passion. Light. He lives his life strongly led by his faith. He is genuinely passionate about helping people and ensuring a better, healthier future for them and without realising it he is a light in many people's lives. - Dr Luke Pendock

Cuan has an incredible ability to relate to people of all ages while providing unique practical guidelines for sustained healthy living - Jabin Lyons

Cuan is one of the most knowledgeable people I know and a true professional at what he does. As a running coach, I cannot work without him - Nick Bester

I believe that healthcare in all forms is a calling which requires the caregiver to always act ethically, professionally, and solely in the interests of the patient at all times. Cuan is a fine example of this, one who treats with knowledge, compassion, grace and a passion for wellness. He practices what he preaches in the way that he lives his life and is a fine example of someone who actively demonstrates true knowledge in his field, compassion and integrity. - Bradley Birkholtz

Having known Cuan from his student years, he was the ever inquisitive and curious student asking a million questions. Cuan has never been able to sit still. He lives and thrives on movement and is now incorporating that into his practice. – Dr Charmaine Korporaal

About the Author

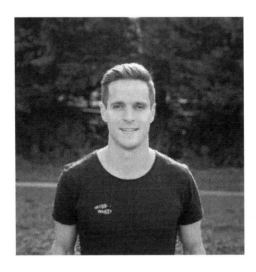

Dr. Cuan Coetzee was born in Durban, South Africa. He is a health coach, accomplished chiropractic physician, and elite athlete, who is considered one of the most prominent advocates for movement as a cure for morbidity.

At 24, he started and trademarked his health and movement coaching brand, MoveMed®, which is also the media platform through which he educates about the benefits of getting moving. He ran his own private practice in East London (SA) for seven years.

At 29, he moved to London and wrote his debut book, WHY MOVEMENT IS MEDICINE. The book is a culmination of his life, his travels, many stories and his clinical and practical experience to date.

The ideas and journaling for this book spanned over a decade, however it was only with his move to London where he had time to put fingers to keyboard. He credits God, his family, and his patients as inspiration for the book.

When not seeing patients in the clinic, or doing outdoor exercise, he is dreaming up the next trail running adventure, surf trip or visit home to see his nephews in South Africa.

As an athlete, he boasts the following personal bests: 400m 48s, 800m 1m55s, 5km 15m30s, 10km 33min, Half marathon 1h19m. Marathon 2h59m.

@cuan33 | g.page/cuan33

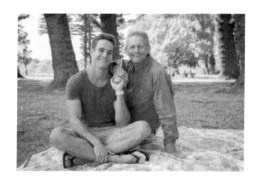

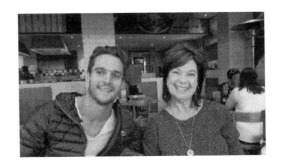

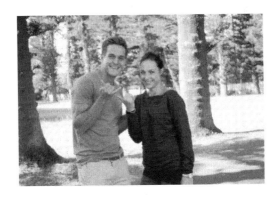

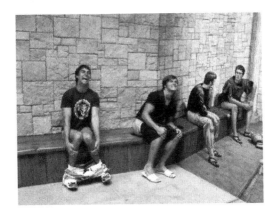

Influential Content

Chapter 1:
Ferrucci L, Simonsick EM. (2006). A little exercise. The journals of gerontology. Series A, Biological sciences and medical sciences, 61(11), 1154–
1156. https://doi.org/10.1093/gerona/61.11.1154.
Philipp LR, Baum GR, Grossberg JA, Ahmad FU. (2016). Baastrup's Disease: An Often Missed Etiology for Back
Pain. Cureus 8(1), 465. https://www.cureus.com/articles/3982-baastrups-disease-an-often-missed-etiology-for-back-pain.
The New Science of Exercise. September 12, 2016 issue of TIME.

Chapter 2:
Ponzio DY, Syed UM, Purcell K, Cooper AM, Maltenfort M, Shaner J, Chen AF. (2018). Low Prevalence of Hip and Knee Arthritis in Active Marathon Runners. The Journal of Bone and Joint Surgery. 100(2), 131-
137. https://pubmed.ncbi.nlm.nih.gov/29342063/
Samborski P, Chmielarz-Czarnocińska A, Grzymisławski M. (2013). Exercise-induced vomiting. Przeglad gastroenterologiczny, 8(6), 396-400. https://doi.org/10.5114/pg.2013.39924
https://results.nyrr.org/
www.strava.com

Chapter 3:
Neef NE, Anwander A, Bütfering C, Schmidt-Samoa C, Friederici AD, Paulus W, Sommer M. (2018). Structural connectivity of right frontal hyperactive areas scales with stuttering severity. Brain. 141(1), 191–
204. https://doi.org/10.1093/ brain/awx316.
Vles GF, Magampa R, Boutall A, Maqungo S. (2017). Primary fusobacterium osteomyelitis and pyomyositis of the thigh in an immunocompetent young adult. S. Afr. j. surg. 55(1), 38-
40. http://www.scielo.org.za/scielo.php?script=sci_arttext&pid=S0038-23612017000100008&lng=en&nrm=iso>.

Basaran R, Kaksi M, Efendioglu M, Onoz M, Balkuv E, Kaner T. (2015). Spinal arachnoid cyst associated with arachnoiditis following subarachnoid haemorrhage in adult patients: A case report and literature review. British Journal of Neurosurgery. 29(2), 285-289, DOI: 10.3109/02688697.2014.976175
https://journal.crossfit.com/

Chapter 5:
The brain-changing benefits of exercise | Wendy Suzuki | Ted Talk | Youtube.com
Sleep is your superpower | Matt Walker | Youtube.com
Alibegovic AC, Sonne MP, Hojbjerre L, Bork-Jensen J, Jacobsen S, Nilsson E, Faerch K, Hiscock NJ, Mortensen B, Friedrichsen M, Stallknecht B, Dela F, Vaag A. (2010). Insulin resistance induced by physical inactivity is associated with multiple transcriptional changes in skeletal muscle in young men. American Journal of Physiology-Endocrinology and Metabolism. 299(5). 752-763. https://journals.physiology.org/doi/pdf/10.1152/ajpendo.0059 0.2009
Lirette LS, Chaiban G, Tolba R, Eissa H. (2014). Coccydynia: An Overview of the Anatomy, Etiology, and Treatment of Coccyx Pain. Ochsner Journal. 14(1), 84-87. https://www.ncbi.nlm.nih.gov/pmc/articles/PMC3963058/pdf/i 1524-5012-14-1-84.pdf

Chapter 6:
Nickell LT, Schucany WG, Opatowsky MJ. (2013). Kummell disease. Proc (Bayl Univ Med Cent). 26(3), 300-301. https://www.ncbi.nlm.nih.gov/pmc/articles/PMC3684306/.
Fuso FA, Dias AL, Letaif OB, Cristante AF, Marcon RM, de Barros TE. (2013). Epidemiological study of cauda equina syndrome. Acta ortopedica brasileira. 21(3), 159-162. https://doi.org/10.1590/S1413-78522013000300006

Chapter 7:
Mad Men Logo. From the TV series Mad Men. Made with Paint 3D

Dimitrov S, Hulteng E, Hong S. (2017). Inflammation and exercise: Inhibition of monocytic intracellular TNF production by acute exercise via β2-adrenergic activation. Brain, Behavior, and Immunity. 61, 60-68. https://doi.org/10.1016/j.bbi.2016.12.017.
Verkhoshansky Y. (1979). Principles of planning speed/strength training program in track athletes. Legaya Athleticka. 8, 8-10.
Luke A, Lazaro RM, Bergeron MF, Keyser L, Benjamin H, Brenner J, d'Hemecourt P, Grady M, Philpott J, Smith A. (2011). Sports-related injuries in youth athletes: is overscheduling a risk factor? Clin J Sport Med. 21(4), 307-14. doi:10.1097/JSM.0b013e3182218f71.
Berdishevsky H. (2016). Outcome of intensive outpatient rehabilitation and bracing in an adult patient with Scheuermann's disease evaluated by radiologic imaging—a case report. Scoliosis. 11(40). https://doi.org/10.1186/s13013-016-0094-7
Kyere KA, Than KD, Wang AC, Rahman SU, Valdivia-Valdivia JM, La Marca F, Park P. (2012). Schmorl's nodes. European spine journal : official publication of the European Spine Society, the European Spinal Deformity Society, and the European Section of the Cervical Spine Research Society. 21(11), 2115-2121. https://doi.org/10.1007/s00586-012-2325-9

Chapter 8:
Dr Robyn Spring conversations between 2013 and 2020
https://www.nhs.uk/conditions/back-pain/.
Fayaz A, Croft P, Langford RM, Donaldson LJ, Jones GT. (2016). Prevalence of chronic pain in the UK: a systematic review and meta-analysis of population studies. BMJ open. 6(6), e010364. https://doi.org/10.1136/bmjopen-2015-010364
Gazit Y, Jacob G, Grahame R. (2016). Ehlers–Danlos Syndrome—Hypermobility Type: A Much Neglected Multisystemic Disorder. Rambam Maimonides Med J. 7(4), e0034. doi:10.5041/RMMJ.10261 review
Alikhan MM, Lohr KM, Driver K. Paget Disease Clinical Presentation.
Medscape. http://emedicine.medscape.com/article/334607-clinical.

Chapter 9:

de la Motte SJ, Lisman P, Gribbin TC, Murphy K, Deuster PA. (2019). Systematic Review of the Association Between Physical Fitness and Musculoskeletal Injury Risk: Part 3-Flexibility, Power, Speed, Balance, and Agility. *J Strength Cond Res*. 33(6), 1723-1735. doi:10.1519/JSC.0000000000002382

Chapter 10:
Mackenzie M. Herzog and Zachary Y. Kerr and Stephen W. Marshall and Erik A. (2019). Epidemiology of Ankle Sprains and Chronic Ankle Instability. Journal of Athletic Training. 54(6), 603-610. https://doi.org/10.4085/1062-6050-447-17
Mazloumi SM, Ebrahimzadeh MH, Kachooei AR. (2014). Evolution in diagnosis and treatment of Legg-Calve-Perthes disease. The archives of bone and joint surgery. 2(2), 86-92. http://abjs.mums.ac.ir/article_3071_ce09c70b9dd0517343986d72549d0359.pdf

Chapter 11:
The Wolf of Wallstreet Logo. From the movie Wolf of Wallstreet. Made with Paint 3D
Milewski MD, Skaggs DL, Bishop GA, et al. (2014). Chronic lack of sleep is associated with increased sports injuries in adolescent athletes. J Pediatr Orthop. 34(2), 129-133. doi:10.1097/BPO.0000000000000151
Bellesi M, Riedner BA, Garcia-Molina GN, Cirelli C, Tononi G. (2014). Enhancement of sleep slow waves: underlying mechanisms and practical consequences. Front Syst Neurosci. 28(8), 208. doi:10.3389/fnsys.2014.00208. PMID: 25389394; PMCID: PMC4211398.
Tononi G, Cirelli C. (2006). Sleep Function and Synaptic Homeostasis. Sleep Med Rev., 10(1), 49-62.
Parker AE, Robb SA, Chambers J, Davidson AC, Evans K, O'Dowd J, Williams AJ, Howard RS. (2005). Analysis of an adult Duchenne muscular dystrophy population, QJM: An International Journal of Medicine. 98(10), 729-736. https://doi.org/10.1093/qjmed/hci113

Chapter 12:

Coetzee CW. (2014). An injury profile of amateur and semi-professional KwaZulu-Natal triathletes. Master's dissertation, Durban University of Technology.
How "normal people" can train like the world's best endurance athletes | Stephen Seiler | TEDx Arendal
Seiler S. (2010). What is Best Practice for Training Intensity and Duration Distribution in Endurance Athletes?. International journal of sports physiology and performance. 5, 276-91.
http://hdl.handle.net/10321/995

Chapter 13:

After watching this, your brain will not be the same | Lara Boyd | TEDx Vancouver | Youtube.com
The most important lesson from 83,000 brain scans | Daniel Amen | TEDx Orange Coast | Youtube.com
2.11 Exercise: Nature's Medicine for Depression and Stress | Dr. Luria | Youtube.com
Blumenthal JA, Babyak MA, Moore KA, et al. (1999). Effects of Exercise Training on Older Patients With Major Depression. Arch Intern Med. 159(19), 2349-356. doi:10.1001/archinte.159.19.2349
Liu-Ambrose T, Nagamatsu LS, Graf P, Beattie BL, Ashe MC, Handy TC. (2010). Resistance training and executive functions: a 12-month randomized controlled trial. *Arch Intern Med.* 170(2):170-178. doi:10.1001/archinternmed.2009.494.
Rehfeld K, Müller P, Aye N, et al. (2017). Dancing or Fitness Sport? The Effects of Two Training Programs on Hippocampal Plasticity and Balance Abilities in Healthy Seniors. *Front Hum Neurosci.* 11, 305. doi:10.3389/fnhum.2017.00305
Akhtar K., Qadri S, Sen Ray P, Sherwani RK. (2014). Cytological diagnosis of chondroblastoma: diagnostic challenge for the cytopathologist. BMJ case reports. bcr2014204178. https://doi.org/10.1136/bcr-2014-204178
Frush TJ, Noyes FR. (2015). Baker's Cyst: Diagnostic and Surgical Considerations. *Sports Health.* 7(4), 359-365. doi:10.1177/1941738113520130
Patel J, Eloy J, Liu JK. (2015). Nelson's syndrome: a review of the clinical manifestations, pathophysiology, and treatment strategies, Neurosurgical Focus FOC. 38(2),

E14. https://thejns.org/focus/view/journals/neurosurg-focus/38/2/article-pE14.xml

"Sertraline Hydrochloride". *Drugs.com*. The American Society of Health-System Pharmacists. Retrieved 24 September 2020.

Chapter 14:

James JE. (2016). Sources of Harm: Prescription Drugs, Surgery, and Infections. The Health of Populations. 133-173. https://doi.org/10.1016/B978-0-12-802812-4.00006-0

Green BN, Johnson CD, Snodgrass J, Smith M, Dunn AS. (2016). Association Between Smoking and Back Pain in a Cross-Section of Adult Americans. Cureus. 8(9), e806. https://doi.org/10.7759/cureus.806

Wu A, Zou F, Cao Y, Xia D, He W, Zhu B, Chen D, Ni W. Wang X, Kwan K. (2017). Lumbar spinal stenosis: an update on the epidemiology, diagnosis and treatment. AME Medical Journal. 2(5). http://amj.amegroups.com/article/view/3837

Schroeder GD, Guyre CA, Vaccaro AR. (2016). The epidemiology and pathophysiology of lumbar disc herniations. Seminars in Spine Surgery. 28(1), 2-7. ISSN 1040-7383. https://doi.org/10.1053/j.semss.2015.08.003.

Fournier JC, DeRubeis RJ, Hollon SD, Dimidjian S, Amsterdam JD, Shelton RC, Fawcett J. (2010). Antidepressant drug effects and depression severity: a patient-level meta-analysis. JAMA. 303(1), 47-53. https://doi.org/10.1001/jama.2009.1943

Kirsch I, Deacon BJ, Huedo-Medina TB, Scoboria A, Moore TJ, Johnson BT. (2008). Initial Severity and Antidepressant Benefits: A Meta-Analysis of Data Submitted to the Food and Drug Administration. PLoS Med. 5(2), e45. https://doi.org/10.1371/journal.pmed.0050045

Johnson CF, Williams B, MacGillivray SA, Dougall NJ, Maxwell M. (2017). 'Doing the right thing': factors influencing GP prescribing of antidepressants and prescribed doses. BMC family practice. 18(1), 72. https://doi.org/10.1186/s12875-017-0643-z

Davies J, Davies D. (2010). Origins and evolution of antibiotic resistance. Microbiology and molecular biology reviews : MMBR. 74(3), 417-433. https://doi.org/10.1128/MMBR.00016-10

Lewis T, Cook J. (2014). Fluoroquinolones and tendinopathy: a guide for athletes and sports clinicians and a systematic review of the literature. Journal of athletic training. 49(3), 422-427. https://doi.org/10.4085/1062-6050-49.2.09

Chapter 15:
Rastogi V, Rawls A, Moore O, et al. (2015). Rare etiology of bow hunter's syndrome and systematic review of literature. J Vasc Interv Neurol. 8(7).
Bogduk N. (2001). Cervicogenic headache: anatomic basis and pathophysiologic mechanisms. Curr Pain Headache Rep. 5(4), 382-386.
Missaghi B. (2004). Sternocleidomastoid syndrome: a case study. J Can Chiropr Assoc. 48(3), 201-205. PMID:17549118; PMCID:PMC1769463.
Simons D, Travell J. (1999). Travell & Simons' myofascial pain and dysfunction: the trigger point manual. Baltimore: Williams & Wilkins.
Fernández-de-las-Peñas C, Alonso-Blanco C, Cuadrado ML, Gerwin RD, Pareja JA. (2006). Trigger points in the suboccipital muscles and forward head posture in tension-type headache. Headache. 46, 454-60. doi:10.1111/j.1526-4610.2006.00288.x
Do TP, Heldarskard GF, Kolding LT, Hvedstrup J, Schytz HW. (2018). Myofascial trigger points in migraine and tension-type headache. J Headache Pain. 19(1), 84. doi:10.1186/s10194-018-0913-8. PMID:30203398; PMCID:PMC6134706.
Oza A, Rajkumar SV. (2015). Waldenstrom macroglobulinemia: prognosis and management. Blood cancer journal. 5(3), e394. https://doi.org/10.1038/bcj.2015.28
Maheshwari PK, Pandey A. (2012). Unusual headaches. Annals of neurosciences. 19(4), 172-176. https://doi.org/10.5214/ans.0972.7531.190409

Chapter 16:
Genetics:
Dean Ornish. Ted Talk 2008 "Your genes are not your fate"
Ferris LT1, Williams JS, Shen CL. (2007). The effect of acute exercise on serum brain-derived neurotrophic factor levels and cognitive function. Med Sci Sports Exerc. 39(4), 728-34.

Rezapour S, Shiravand M, Mardani M. (2018). Epigenetic changes due to physical activity. Biotechnol Appl Biochem. 65(6):761-767.

Chaya S, Zampoli M, Gray D, et al. (2018). The First Case of Riboflavin Transporter Deficiency in sub-Saharan Africa. *Semin Pediatr Neurol.* 26, 10-14. doi:10.1016/j.spen.2017.03.002

Fasting:

Pinto AP, Vieira TS, Marafon BB, et al. (2020). The Combination of Fasting, Acute Resistance Exercise, and Protein Ingestion Led to Different Responses of Autophagy Markers in Gastrocnemius and Liver Samples. *Nutrients.* 12(3):641. doi:10.3390/nu12030641

Heilbronn LK, Smith SR, Martin CK, Anton SD, Ravussin E. (2005). Alternate-day fasting in nonobese subjects: effects on body weight, body composition, and energy metabolism, The American Journal of Clinical Nutrition. 81(1), 69-73. https://doi.org/10.1093/ajcn/81.1.69

Hartman ML, Veldhuis JD, Johnson ML, Lee MM, Alberti KG, Samojlik E, Thorner MO. (1992). Augmented growth hormone (GH) secretory burst frequency and amplitude mediate enhanced GH secretion during a two-day fast in normal men, The Journal of Clinical Endocrinology & Metabolism. 74(4), 757-765. https://doi.org/10.1210/jcem.74.4.1548337

Alirezaei M, Kemball CC, Flynn CT, Wood MR, Whitton JL, Kiosses WB. (2010). Short-term fasting induces profound neuronal autophagy. Autophagy. 6(6), 702-710. https://doi.org/10.4161/auto.6.6.12376

Martin B, Mattson MP, Maudsley S. (2006). Caloric restriction and intermittent fasting: two potential diets for successful brain aging. Ageing research reviews. 5(3), 332-353. https://doi.org/10.1016/j.arr.2006.04.002

Zhu Y, Yan Y, Gius DR, Vassilopoulos A. (2013). Metabolic regulation of Sirtuins upon fasting and the implication for cancer. Current opinion in oncology. 25(6), 630-636. https://doi.org/10.1097/01.cco.0000432527.49984.a3

Chapter 17:

How much exercise is too much? | Tim Noakes | TEDx Cape Town | Youtube.com

Lampe JW. Dairy products and cancer. *J Am Coll Nutr.* 2011;30(5 Suppl 1):464S-70S. doi:10.1080/07315724.2011.10719991

Waterlogged: The Serious Problem of Overhydration in Endurance Sports: Amazon.co.uk: Tim Noakes, Timothy Noakes: 8601234621140: Books.

Lustig RH. (2013). Fructose: It's "Alcohol Without the Buzz", Advances in Nutrition. 4(2), 226-235. https://doi.org/10.3945/an.112.002998

Noakes T, Sboros M. (2017). Lore of nutrition: challenging conventional dietary beliefs. https://www.overdrive.com/search?q=CA542DF1-0C90-474B-BCD5-0736C776FFBC.

Sung B, Prasad S, Gupta SC, Patchva S, Aggarwal BB. (2012). Chapter 3 - Regulation of Inflammation-Mediated Chronic Diseases by Botanicals. Advances in Botanical Research, Academic Press. 62, 57-132. https://doi.org/10.1016/B978-0-12-394591-4.00003-9.

Seidelmann SB, Claggett B, Cheng S, et al. (2018). Dietary carbohydrate intake and mortality: a prospective cohort study and meta-analysis. *Lancet Public Health.* 3(9), e419-e428. doi:10.1016/S2468-2667(18)30135-X

Michaëlsson K, Wolk A, Langenskiöld S., Basu S, Warensjö Lemming E, Melhus H, Byberg L. (2014). Milk intake and risk of mortality and fractures in women and men: cohort studies. BMJ (Clinical research ed.). 349, g6015. https://doi.org/10.1136/bmj.g6015

Vasconcelos IM, Oliveira JT. (2004). Antinutritional properties of plant lectins. Toxicon. 44(4), 385-403. https://doi.org/10.1016/j.toxicon.2004.05.005

Aune D, Navarro Rosenblatt DA, Chan DS, et al. (2015). Dairy products, calcium, and prostate cancer risk: a systematic review and meta-analysis of cohort studies. *Am J Clin Nutr.* 101(1), 87-117. doi:10.3945/ajcn.113.067157

Kato-Kataoka A, Nishida K, Takada M, et al. (2016). Fermented Milk Containing Lactobacillus casei Strain Shirota Preserves the Diversity of the Gut Microbiota and Relieves Abdominal Dysfunction in Healthy Medical Students Exposed to Academic

Stress. *Appl Environ Microbiol.* 82(12), 3649-3658. doi:10.1128/AEM.04134-15

Akbari S, Rasouli-Ghahroudi AA. (2018). Vitamin K and Bone Metabolism: A Review of the Latest Evidence in Preclinical Studies. *Biomed Res Int.* 2018; 2018:4629383. Published 2018 Jun 27. doi:10.1155/2018/4629383

Chapter 18:

Pappolla MA, Manchikanti L, Andersen CR, Greig NH, Ahmed F, Fang X, et al. (2019) Is insulin resistance the cause of fibromyalgia? A preliminary report. PLoS ONE 14(5): e0216079. https://doi.org/10.1371/journal.pone.0216079

Hart RP, Wade JB, Martelli MF. (2003). Cognitive impairment in patients with chronic pain: the significance of stress. Current Pain and Headache Reports. 7(2), 116-126. doi:10.1007/s11916-003-0021-5.

Bruehl S, Burns JW, Chung OY, Chont M. (2009). Pain-related effects of trait anger expression: neural substrates and the role of endogenous opioid mechanisms. Neuroscience and Biobehavioral Reviews. 33(3), 475-491. doi: 10.1016/j.neubiorev.2008.12.003.

Fields HL, Martin JB. (2005). Harrison's Principles of Internal Medicine. 16th ed. New York: McGraw-Hill. 71-6. http://www.medicaldictionary.thefreedictionary.com.

Burket LW, Greenberg MS, Glick M. Burkett's Textbook of Oral Medicine. 10th ed. Philadelphia, PA: Lippincott.

Bennett CR. Monheim's Local Anesthesia and Pain Control in Dental Practice. 7th ed. St. Louis, MO: C.V. Mosby; 1984.

McCaffery M, Pasero C. (1999). Pain: A Clinical Manual. 2nd ed. St. Louis: Mosby, Inc.

Kumar KH, Elavarasi P. (2016). Definition of pain and classification of pain disorders. J Adv Clin Res Insights. 3, 87-90.

Rathmacher JA, Fuller JC Jr, Baier SM, Abumrad NN, Angus HF, Sharp RL. (2012). Adenosine-5'-triphosphate (ATP) supplementation improves low peak muscle torque and torque fatigue during repeated high intensity exercise sets. J Int Soc Sports Nutr. 9(1), 48. doi:10.1186/1550-2783-9-48

Mu Q, Kirby J, Reilly CM, Luo XM. (2017). Leaky Gut As a Danger Signal for Autoimmune Diseases. Front. Immunol. 8, 598. doi:10.3389/fimmu.2017.00598

Garland EL. (2012). Pain processing in the human nervous system: a selective review of nociceptive and biobehavioral pathways. Primary care. 39(3), 561-571. https://doi.org/10.1016/j.pop.2012.06.013

Chapter 19:
Sakallaris BR, MacAllister L, Voss M, Smith K, Jonas WB. (2015). Optimal healing environments. Global advances in health and medicine. 4(3), 40-45. https://doi.org/10.7453/gahmj.2015.043
Cui K. Li W. Liu X, et al. (2016). Effect of cervical manipulation on autonomic nervous function in healthy volunteers. Journal of Acupuncture and Tuina Science. 4, 267-270.
McCorry LK. (2007). Physiology of the autonomic nervous system. Am J Pharm Educ. 71(4), 78. doi:10.5688/aj710478.
Rome PL. (2009). Neurovertebral Influence upon the Autonomic Nervous System: Some of the Somato-autonomic Evidence to Date. Chiropractic Journal of Australia. 39(1), 2-17. https://search.informit.com.au/documentSummary;dn=381380 637326858;res=IELHEA.
Waxenbaum JA, Varacallo M. (2019). Anatomy, Autonomic Nervous System. https://www.ncbi.nlm.nih.gov/books/NBK539845/
Welch A, Boone R. (2008). Sympathetic and parasympathetic responses to specific diversified adjustments to chiropractic vertebral subluxations of the cervical and thoracic spine. Journal of chiropractic medicine. 7(3), 86-93. https://doi.org/10.1016/j.jcm.2008.04.001
Salkind, N. J. (2010). Encyclopedia of research design (Vols. 1-0). Thousand Oaks, CA: SAGE Publications, Inc. doi: 10.4135/9781412961288

Chapter 20:
Callendar A. (2007). The mechanistic/ vitalistic dualism of chiropractic and general systems theory: Daniel D. Palmer and Ludwig von Bertalanffy. J Chiropr Humanit. 14, 1-21.
Palmer D. (1910). Portland Printing House; Portland, OR. The science, art, and philosophy of chiropractic.

Wang H, Yu M, Ochani M, et al. (2003). Nicotinic acetylcholine receptor alpha7 subunit is an essential regulator of inflammation. Nature. 421, 384-388.

Jahan F, Nanji K, Qidwai W, Qasim R. (2012). Fibromyalgia syndrome: an overview of pathophysiology, diagnosis and management. Oman medical journal. 27(3), 192-195. https://doi.org/10.5001/omj.2012.44

Cohen H. (2017). Controversies and challenges in fibromyalgia: a review and a proposal. Therapeutic advances in musculoskeletal disease. 9(5), 115-127. https://doi.org/10.1177/1759720X17699199

ٮ

Made in the USA
Columbia, SC
05 January 2024

29934732R10245